MAP KEY

Other titles in this series

THE BEST IN TENT CAMPING

A GUIDE FOR CAR CAMPERS WHO HATE RVs,
CONCRETE SLABS, AND LOUD PORTABLE STEREOS

ILLINOIS

JOHN SCHIRLE

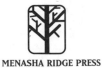

MENASHA RIDGE PRESS

BIRMINGHAM, ALABAMA

Copyright © 2009 by John Schirle

Printed in the United States of America
Published by Menasha Ridge Press
Distributed by Publishers Group West
First edition, first printing

Library of Congress Cataloging-in-Publication Data
Schirle, John.
    The best in tent camping, Illinois : a guide for car campers who hate RVs, concrete slabs, and
loud portable stereos / by John Schirle.
    p. cm.
    Includes index.
    ISBN-13: 978-0-89732-643-8
    ISBN-10: 0-89732-643-1
    1. Camping—Illinois—Guidebooks. 2. Camp sites, facilities, etc.—Illinois—Guidebooks.
3. Illinois—Guidebooks. I. Title.
    GV191.42.I3S33 2009
    917.77304'44—dc22

                                2009011261

Cover and text design by Ian Szymkowiak, Palace Press International, Inc.
Cover photo by Ted Villaire
Cartography by Steve Jones and John Schirle
Indexing by Ann Cassar

Menasha Ridge Press
P.O. Box 43673
Birmingham, Alabama 35243
www.menasharidge.com

TABLE OF CONTENTS

SOUTHERN ILLINOIS

THE BEST ILLINOIS CAMPGROUNDS

BEST FOR FISHING

5. LOUD THUNDER FOREST PRESERVE
14. SILOAM SPRINGS STATE PARK
15. JIM EDGAR PANTHER CREEK STATE FISH & WILDLIFE AREA
22. BEAVER DAM STATE PARK
23. RAMSEY LAKE STATE PARK
24. EAGLE CREEK STATE PARK
25. WALNUT POINT STATE PARK
29. SAM DALE LAKE STATE FISH & WILDLIFE AREA
34. WAYNE FITZGERRELL STATE PARK
41. LITTLE GRASSY CAMPGROUND
42. DEVILS KITCHEN CAMPGROUND

BEST FOR HIKING

1. APPLE RIVER CANYON STATE PARK
5. LOUD THUNDER FOREST PRESERVE
11. SAND RIDGE STATE FOREST
19. KICKAPOO STATE PARK
38. PINE HILLS CAMPGROUND
43. FERNE CLYFFE STATE PARK
44. RED BUD CAMPGROUND
47. PHARAOH CAMPGROUND/ GARDEN OF THE GODS RECREATION AREA

BEST FOR CANOEING

3. SUGAR RIVER FOREST PRESERVE
5. LOUD THUNDER FOREST PRESERVE
7. CHANNAHON AND GEBHARD WOODS STATE PARKS
18. MIDDLE FORK STATE FISH & WILDLIFE AREA
19. KICKAPOO STATE PARK

BEST FOR CYCLING/MOUNTAIN-BIKING

5. LOUD THUNDER FOREST PRESERVE
6. JOHNSON-SAUK TRAIL STATE RECREATION AREA (NEARBY)
7. CHANNAHON AND GEBHARD WOODS STATE PARKS
12. COMLARA PARK

(continued)

15. JIM EDGAR PANTHER CREEK STATE FISH & WILDLIFE AREA
19. KICKAPOO STATE PARK

BEST FOR SWIMMING

12. COMLARA PARK
16. FRIENDS CREEK CONSERVATION AREA (NEARBY)
24. EAGLE CREEK STATE PARK (NEARBY)
28. STEPHEN A. FORBES STATE RECREATION AREA
29. SAM DALE LAKE STATE FISH & WILDLIFE AREA
34. WAYNE FITZGERRELL STATE PARK (NEARBY)
45. DIXON SPRINGS STATE PARK (POOL)
48. PINE RIDGE CAMPGROUND/ POUNDS HOLLOW RECREATION AREA

BEST FOR FAMILIES WITH KIDS

12. COMLARA PARK
20. FOREST GLEN COUNTY PRESERVE
34. WAYNE FITZGERRELL STATE PARK
40. GIANT CITY STATE PARK
45. DIXON SPRINGS STATE PARK

BEST FOR BEAUTY

1. APPLE RIVER CANYON STATE PARK
22. BEAVER DAM STATE PARK
35. HAMILTON COUNTY STATE FISH & WILDLIFE AREA
43. FERNE CLYFFE STATE PARK
47. PHARAOH CAMPGROUND/ GARDEN OF THE GODS RECREATION AREA

BEST FOR PRIVACY

4. MARENGO RIDGE FOREST PRESERVE
11. SAND RIDGE STATE FOREST
17. LODGE PARK
39. TRAIL OF TEARS STATE FOREST
43. FERNE CLYFFE STATE PARK

THE BEST
ILLINOIS
CAMPGROUNDS
(CONTINUED)

BEST FOR SPACIOUSNESS

3. SUGAR RIVER FOREST PRESERVE
15. JIM EDGAR PANTHER CREEK STATE FISH & WILDLIFE AREA
23. RAMSEY LAKE STATE PARK
29. SAM DALE LAKE STATE FISH & WILDLIFE AREA
39. TRAIL OF TEARS STATE FOREST

BEST FOR QUIET

9. WOODFORD COUNTY STATE FISH & WILDLIFE AREA
11. SAND RIDGE STATE FOREST
37. TURKEY BAYOU CAMPGROUND
39. TRAIL OF TEARS STATE FOREST
47. PHARAOH CAMPGROUND/ GARDEN OF THE GODS RECREATION AREA

BEST FOR SECURITY

4. MARENGO RIDGE FOREST PRESERVE
22. BEAVER DAM STATE PARK
23. RAMSEY LAKE STATE PARK
28. STEPHEN A. FORBES STATE RECREATION AREA

BEST FOR CLEANLINESS

2. LAKE LE-AQUA-NA STATE PARK
12. COMLARA PARK
15. JIM EDGAR PANTHER CREEK STATE FISH & WILDLIFE AREA
16. FRIENDS CREEK CONSERVATION AREA
35. HAMILTON COUNTY STATE FISH & WILDLIFE AREA

ACKNOWLEDGMENTS

A huge thanks to all the personnel with the Illinois Department of Natural Resources, the U.S. Forest Service, the U.S. Fish and Wildlife Service, and the various county conservation districts and forest preserves across Illinois who provided so much help as I researched this book. They patiently answered my questions, responded to my phone calls and emails, and even gave me guided tours around their properties. Illinois has tremendous natural beauty, but it is carefully maintained and kept accessible only through the often-unsung efforts of these folks.

Thanks also to my caving buddies in the Near Normal Grotto of the National Speleological Society, who not only provided me with excellent campground recommendations but also put up with hardly seeing me for more than a year. (Honest guys, now that this is done, I'm ready to head underground again!).

Thanks to Mary Handley, who taught me at Stephen Decatur High School to delight in writing.

Thanks to my co-workers at the Decatur Public Library Children's Department, who graciously juggled schedules to allow me time to travel and camp.

Thanks to my good friend Mark Sturgell, who not only encouraged me along the way but also painstakingly proofread every campground profile, helping me see what I had missed.

Thanks to the folk at Menasha Ridge Press, including Molly Merkle, Holly Cross, and all the others behind the scenes, who patiently worked with this first-time author to create what I hope will be a helpful addition to an excellent series.

Thanks above all to God, who crafted the prairies, forests, canyons, bluffs, rivers, and lakes that are Illinois today and gave them to us to care for and enjoy.

PREFACE

If you've picked up this book, I expect that for you, like me, camping is not just overnight lodging—it's part of the entire outdoor experience. You want to pitch your tent on soft grass surrounded by woods, to be lulled to sleep by the sound of a nearby creek rippling between its banks, to wake to watch the sunrise across the lake. (Just reading these words, you've probably pulled out your calendar to find your next free weekend.) For years I've searched the Midwest for such perfect spots, and found that Web sites and even most books don't tell the whole story. That's why I was delighted to stumble across Menasha Ridge Press's *The Best in Tent Camping: Missouri and the Ozarks,* which accompanied me on several wonderful trips. I was even more delighted when Menasha Ridge asked if I'd be willing to author this volume on my home state of Illinois.

Exploring Illinois for this book has been fun. From north to south and east to west, it's been an adventure, discovering so many wonderful rivers to canoe, lakes to fish, trails to hike, woods to wander, and quiet places to camp. I knew some places I wanted to include from the start (like my all-time favorite, Ferne Clyffe State Park), but as I traversed the state, first by phone and Internet and then by car, I uncovered more and more fascinating and diverse wild places that I had to share. Some were places I'd long wanted to visit, such as Apple River Canyon State Park to the northwest, with its bubbling creeks and steep ravines. Others were completely off my radar, surprises that I stumbled across, such as virtually unvisited McCully Heritage Project to the southwest or Lodge Park along the Sangamon River, barely 30 miles from my hometown. I kept discovering new places—the research was so much fun that the hardest part was to stop exploring and start writing!

Knowing that "ideal campsite" conjures different images for each of us, I've tried to include a variety of campgrounds. All have non-electric sites in a natural setting, and most either don't attract RVs or have separate RV and tent areas. Some have few or no amenities but offer secluded sites where you're almost sure to be by yourself. Others offer a shower building, restaurant, and store. At some you can fish, hike, boat, bike, swim, or even go rock-climbing; others are perfect for simply relaxing. Many are near other natural or historic sites, which I've included. Among them, I hope you will find places that are a perfect fit.

I hope I've been thorough, and doubt I've been exhaustive. I'm sure tucked away in some corner of the state—or perhaps just a few miles down the road—is yet another camping getaway, kept secret by the few who visit it year after year. If you encounter some special place that deserves to be included in a future edition of this book (and don't mind sharing the secret!), let me know at **illinoiscamper@gmail.com.**

Meanwhile, throw your gear in the car and head out to explore the Prairie State!

ABOUT THE AUTHOR

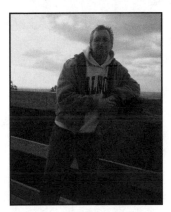

John Schirle was raised in central Illinois and has been back in his home state since 1993. Since his college days, he has loved getting away in the outdoors—camping, hiking, canoeing, and, more recently, caving. As a result he has spent countless hours scouring the region for the ever-elusive ideal tent-camping getaway. His personal goal for some years has been to visit every single state park in Illinois (he hasn't yet achieved this goal, but he's a lot closer now!). Over the years he has been a Bible translator in central Africa, a college professor, camp program director, and is currently a children's librarian and writing tutor in his hometown of Decatur, Illinois. And he's the only Menasha Ridge author who speaks Congolese Swahili.

INTRODUCTION

THE OVERVIEW MAP AND OVERVIEW-MAP KEY

Use the overview map on the inside front cover to assess the exact location of each campground. The campground's number appears not only on the overview map but also on the map key facing the overview map, in the table of contents, and on the profile's first page.

The book is organized by region, as indicated in the table of contents. A map legend that details the symbols found on the campground layout maps appears on the inside back cover.

CAMPGROUND-LAYOUT MAPS

Each profile contains a detailed campground layout map that provides an overhead look at campground sites, internal roads, facilities, and other key items. Each park entrance's GPS coordinates are included with each profile.

GPS CAMPGROUND-ENTRANCE COORDINATES

Readers can easily access all campgrounds in this book by using the directions given and the overview map, which shows at least one major road leading into the area. But for those who enjoy using the latest GPS technology to navigate, the necessary data has been provided. To collect accurate map data, each park entrance was recorded with a handheld GPS unit. Data collected was then downloaded and plotted onto a digital USGS topo map. Each profile includes the GPS coordinates in two formats: latitude/longitude and UTM. Latitude/longitude coordinates tell you where you are by locating a point west (longitude) of the 0° meridian line that passes through Greenwich, England, and north or south (latitude) of the 0° line that belts the Earth, the Equator.

The UTM coordinates index a specific point using a grid method. The survey datum used to arrive at the coordinates is WGS84. For readers who own a GPS unit, whether handheld or onboard a vehicle, the Universal Transverse Mercator (UTM) coordinates provided with each campground description may be entered into the GPS unit. Just make sure your GPS unit is set to navigate using the UTM system in conjunction with WGS84 datum.

UTM COORDINATES: ZONE, EASTING, AND NORTHING

Within the UTM coordinates box in each campground description, there are three numbers labeled zone, easting, and northing. Here is an example from the Apple River Canyon State Park profile:

Zone   15T
Easting   0742552
Northing   4703831

The UTM zone number (15) refers to one of the 60 vertical zones of a map using the UTM projection. Each zone is 6 wide. The zone letter (T) refers to one of the 20 horizontal zones that span from 80° South to 84° North. The easting number (0742552) indicates in meters how far east the point is from the zero value, which runs north-south through Greenwich, England. Increasing easting coordinates on a topo map or on your GPS screen indicate you are moving east; decreasing easting coordinates indicate you are moving west. Since lines of longitude converge at the poles, they are not parallel as lines of latitude are. In the Northern Hemisphere, the northing number (4703831) indicates in meters how far you are from the equator. Above the equator, northing coordinates increase by 1,000 meters between each parallel line of latitude (east-west lines). On a topo map or GPS receiver, increasing northing numbers indicate you are traveling north; decreasing northing coordinates indicate you are traveling south.

THE RATING SYSTEM

The campgrounds in this book are rated on a five-star system. A rating of five stars is wonderful, and one star is acceptable. Though these ratings are subjective, they're still excellent guidelines for finding a good camping experience for you and your companions. Some campgrounds have a low rating in one or two areas but are still worth visiting for other reasons. In parks or forests where there are both tent and RV campgrounds, I've rated the tent campground. In places with multiple tent campgrounds, the rating is an average—read the profile for more details.

BEAUTY All of the campgrounds in this guide are either in or near beautiful, natural settings, and in each profile I've endeavored to describe those features. Some of the campgrounds themselves are scenic—on a lakeshore, riverside, or bluff top—while others are more ordinary but near places worth seeing. My rating for beauty focuses primarily on the campground itself.

PRIVACY I'm a camping isolationist, so this one's important to me. Campgrounds with sites spaced well apart and trees and brush between them provide a greater sense of seclusion and earned a higher rating. Others rate high not so much because of site layout but because the campground gets limited use, so you're likely to have few or no neighbors.

SPACIOUSNESS Some folk are content with a small clearing, just big enough to pitch a tent, while others want lots of room to spread out, camp with friends, and set up all their gear. The more spacious sites provide open grassy areas suitable for several tents.

QUIET Campgrounds away from highway and city noise rated higher, as did those that are generally less busy or tend to attract folks looking for quiet. Campgrounds with an onsite ranger or nearby campground host are also usually quieter, since rowdy groups avoid them or are quickly dealt with. Of course nothing can predict when a single noisy neighbor will camp next to you, but if a particular campground was known as a place for parties, I removed it from consideration.

SECURITY I've found Illinois' established campgrounds to be generally safe and secure. Most state- and county-managed campgrounds, and some national forest ones, have rangers who regularly patrol the area, and many have on-site campground hosts during the regular camping season. A few even have a check-in station at the campground entrance to control access. These all received a "4" or "5" rating. The more remote, primitive campgrounds don't have on-site security, but they're also places where few come, and you're less likely to run into opportunistic crime.

Obviously, campground security is relative. When you're living in a tent, there's little to protect your property from unwanted intrusion, and certain precautions are wise. When I'm away from my campsite, the important stuff is either in my backpack or locked in the car. When I'm camping by myself, I carry a charged cell phone and make certain someone back home knows my plans.

CLEANLINESS Every campground I've included was relatively clean and well maintained—trash was picked up, campsites mowed, and water spigots functional. Those that ranked highest obviously go the extra mile to keep restrooms and shower buildings spotless, brush trimmed, even fire pits regularly scooped out. The only "3" rating went to a campground where I saw evidence of old trash, not just what might have been left by the previous occupant.

STATE PARKS

About two-thirds of the campgrounds I've included are managed by the Illinois Department of Natural Resources (IDNR). These include any labeled State Parks, State Recreation Areas, State Forests, and State Fish & Wildlife Areas. (And if you're not sure what category a particular spot is, don't worry, sometimes the IDNR isn't either—the road sign may say "state recreation area," while the official Web site calls it a "state fish & wildlife area," and the ranger will answer the phone with "state park.")

Though the IDNR fees listed are applicable to most campers, certain discounts are available for Illinois residents who are seniors, disabled, disabled veterans, or former POWs. Discounts vary depending on the day of the week and class of campsite. Check **www.dnr.state.il.us/lands/Landmgt/Programs/Camping/fees.htm** for details. Note that the state has proposed adding a vehicle charge for visiting state parks: $5 per vehicle per day or $25 for an annual pass ($35 for out-of-state vehicles). This may be enacted sometime in 2009.

Unfortunately, in recent years the state has cut IDNR's budget and staff, so some services and operating hours have been reduced. The bottom line: when calling or visiting a park office, if you don't find someone there or get an immediate response, be patient. In all the state parks, there are fewer personnel wearing more hats.

SHAWNEE NATIONAL FOREST

The only national forest in Illinois, the Shawnee has more than 275,000 acres of hiking trails and backcountry camping, as well as climbing spots, equestrian trails, and rivers and streams for fishing. Six of the campgrounds in this book are on national forest land.

In addition, primitive camping is allowed on national forest land outside the boundaries of developed campgrounds and picnic areas. Camping is not allowed within designated natural areas, research natural areas, within 150 feet of a municipal water source, or within a quarter mile of a developed campground or picnic area. There is no fee for camping in general forest areas; however, a maximum of 14 days continuous use applies. If you do camp outside a developed campground, be sure you follow all regulations and recommendations for fires and waste disposal. Check **www.fs.fed.us/r9/forests/shawnee/recreation/rogs/ generalcampingpicnic.pdf** for general information.

FIRST-AID KIT

A useful first-aid kit may contain more items than you might think necessary. These are just the basics. Prepackaged kits in waterproof bags (Atwater Carey and Adventure Medical make them) are available. As a preventive measure, take along sunscreen and insect repellent. Even though quite a few items are listed here, they pack down into a small space:

Ace bandages or Spenco joint wraps

Adhesive bandages, such as Band-Aids

Antibiotic ointment (Neosporin or the generic equivalent)

Antiseptic or disinfectant, such as Betadine or hydrogen peroxide

Aspirin or acetaminophen

Benadryl or the generic equivalent, diphenhydramine (in case of allergic reactions)

Butterfly-closure bandages

Comb and tweezers (for removing ticks from your skin)

Emergency poncho

Epinephrine in a prefilled syringe (for people known to have severe allergic reactions to such things as bee stings)

Gauze (one roll)

Gauze compress pads (six 4 x 4 inch pads)

LED flashlight or headlamp

Matches or pocket lighter

Moleskin/Spenco "Second Skin"

Pocketknife or multipurpose tool

Waterproof first-aid tape

Whistle (it's more effective in signaling rescuers than your voice)

ANIMAL AND PLANT HAZARDS

RACCOONS Most wooded areas in Illinois are home to at least some raccoons, which have learned to take advantage of the buffet of foodstuffs we regularly leave out for their enjoyment. I've seen industrious raccoons break into locked coolers and crawl through barely opened car windows to get to scraps of food. To avoid their nocturnal visits:

- Never have food—not even candy, gum, soft drinks, or beer—in your tent.

- Promptly dispose of all garbage with any trace of food on it. If an enclosed trash container is not available, put the garbage sack in a closed vehicle for the night.

- Wipe up or pick up any spilled food.

If you've been cooking meat, raccoons' inquisitive noses may draw them to your campsite, but if you've disposed of everything, let them sniff around and they'll soon determine there's nothing left and wander off.

TICKS Ticks like to hang out in the brush that grows around campsites and along trails. They're most numerous during hot summer months, but you should be tick-aware throughout the year. Two varieties are prevalent in Illinois, dog ticks and deer ticks; the latter may be so tiny you'll have to look carefully to spot them. You may see them on shoes, socks, or hats, and they can take several hours to actually latch on. Both varieties may carry disease, but it requires several hours of actual attachment before it can be transmitted.

If you're going to be hiking where ticks are prevalent, the best prevention is to wear light-colored clothes (so you can see the ticks more readily), long pants tucked into your socks, closed shoes, and an insect repellent with DEET. Check yourself visually several times a day and your whole body carefully at least once a day. Ticks like to migrate to warm, dark places like the back of the knee, inside the thighs, under the waistband or sock elastic, or in the belly button or armpit. Ticks that haven't attached are easily removed but not easily killed. If you pick off a tick in the woods, just toss it aside. If you find one on your body at camp, toss it into the toilet or fire (otherwise it may find you again). For ticks that have attached, removal with tweezers is best. Grasp the tick behind the head as close to the skin surface as possible and pull straight back with a slow steady force, avoiding crushing the tick's body. Thoroughly disinfect the bite site. Practically all tick bites will result in some local redness and itching, but that doesn't mean you've contracted a disease.

MOSQUITOES Although it's not a common occurrence, individuals can become infected with the West Nile virus by being bitten by an infected mosquito. Culex mosquitoes, the primary varieties that can transmit West Nile virus to humans, thrive in urban rather than natural areas. Most people infected with West Nile virus have no symptoms of illness, but some may become ill, usually 3 to 15 days after being bitten.

In Illinois, summer is the time thought to be the highest risk period for West Nile virus. At this time of the year—and any time you expect mosquitoes to be buzzing around—you may want to wear protective clothing, such as long sleeves, long pants, and socks. Loose-fitting, light-colored clothing is best. Spray clothing with insect repellent. Follow the instructions on the repellent and take extra care with children.

EMERALD ASH BORER The emerald ash borer (Agrilus planipennis) is an exotic insect, native to Asia, which currently threatens ash trees in the Great Lakes region. The pest has been found in northeastern and central Illinois and can be spread inadvertently in infested firewood. It is therefore illegal to transport firewood out of any of 21 currently quarantined counties to elsewhere in the state—and discouraged to do so elsewhere. By following some simple rules, you can help prevent the spread of these destructive insects.

- Purchase aged firewood near your campsite location; don't bring it from home. Many parks sell firewood, often delivered right to your site, and it is often available from vendors just outside the parks.
- Firewood purchased at or near your destination should be used during your camping trip; don't take it to another destination.
- Buy wood that has no bark or loose bark (a sign the wood is very dry). This will reduce the chances of infestation while also making your fire easier to start.

For more information, visit **www.illinoiseab.com.**

POISON IVY Recognizing poison ivy and avoiding contact with it is the most effective way to prevent the itchy rash this plant causes. In Illinois, poison ivy can be a small ground plant or climbing vine, with leaflets in clusters of three. The leaves vary in shape, but in Illinois the two outer leaves typically have a single large lobe on the outside edge and not the inside, looking like a mitten.

Urushiol, an oil in the plant, is responsible for the rash and may be present even in the dead or leafless vine. You can get the rash by direct contact with the plant or by later touching shoes, clothing, hiking gear, or even pets on which the oil has rubbed off. As soon after contact as possible, washing the affected skin with alcohol, soap, and water can prevent the rash from developing. If you know you get the rash easily (as I do), always wear long pants when hiking through underbrush and carry an alcohol-based hand sanitizer and a washcloth along with your drinking water. Be sure to eventually wash off shoes and anything else that may have the oil on it.

If you are exposed to poison ivy, raised lines or blisters will usually appear within 12 hours (but sometimes much later), accompanied by a terrible itch. Refrain from scratching because it can cause infection, but it won't spread the rash, as is commonly believed. Wash and dry the area thoroughly. Various over-the-counter products will alleviate the symptoms until it heals on its own. In worse cases, a doctor can prescribe treatment.

TIPS FOR A HAPPY CAMPING TRIP

- **DO SOME HOMEWORK.** Since you're reading this book, I expect that you, like me, prefer to research before traveling. I want to know all there is to see in the area, trails to hike, historic sites, museums, even nearby elephant graves (see the Delabar State Park profile!). I may not choose to visit them all, but knowing the options helps me plan. Check the resources in Appendix A and the Internet. Remember, though, that even official Web sites aren't always regularly updated. I found a few campground Web sites that contained information that hadn't been correct for several years.

- **CALL AHEAD.** There are times you just throw the gear in the car and hit the road, but whenever possible call at least a week before you plan to camp. The details in this book were correct in 2008, but fees go up, office hours change, and any number of unforeseen events can close campgrounds or limit services. Don't just ask "Are you open?" Be specific. One park I visited assured me over the phone that the campgrounds were open, but on arrival I discovered that the walk-in area I specifically wanted had been closed for two years.

  Confirm any details that are important to you: "Is the beach open?" "How are the bass biting?" "What's the condition of the mountain biking trail?" Ask if there are any local events that would attract a larger-than-usual crowd during your visit. Double-check the driving directions—rural roads may temporarily close due to flooding or other circumstances.

- **PICK YOUR CAMPING BUDDIES WISELY.** Make sure you're all on the same page regarding expectations of difficulty, sleeping arrangements, food requirements, and activity plans. If you want to hike while your friend would rather fish, that can work, as long as you've communicated in advance. If he wants showers and flush toilets but you plan to backpack, that may not work. If camping with family, select a campground that will make everyone comfortable. Many state park campgrounds offer primitive sites, RV sites, and air-conditioned cabins all within a short walk of each other.

- **JUST SAY "NO" TO HOLIDAYS.** Most campgrounds are busiest over the Memorial Day, July 4th, Labor Day, and sometimes Columbus Day holidays. Unless your annual family campout is one of those weekends, avoid camping then. If you must, there are a few campgrounds in the book where sites are so spread out (such as Trail of Tears State Forest) that you can still find relative seclusion.

If possible, arrange your camping trips for midweek, when traffic is lighter. The only down-side is that special programs (guided hikes, live music, historic building tours, hayrides, etc.) at some parks are often only scheduled for weekends, when more people are there to participate.

- **DRESS APPROPRIATELY FOR THE SEASON AND YOUR ACTIVITIES.** In the Midwest, you'll often hear: "If you don't like the weather, wait an hour." It may be warm and sunny when you leave home on a summer afternoon but turn cold and wet by the time you bed down at your campsite. Bring extra clothes, layers of clothes, and plan for extremes. If you'll be hiking, bring appropriate, comfortable, and sturdy footwear.

- **PITCH YOUR TENT ON A LEVEL SURFACE,** preferably one that is covered with leaves, pine straw, or grass. If rain is possible, make sure the site is not lower than the surrounding area and prone to flooding. Do a little site maintenance first, such as picking up small rocks and sticks that can dam-age the tent and make sleep uncomfortable. Pitch your tent on a tarp to keep out ground moisture and to protect the tent floor. Look up as well and check for standing dead or storm-damaged trees. These may have loose or broken limbs that can fall at any time.

- **TAKE A SLEEPING PAD OR AIR MATTRESS** if you are not used to sleeping on the ground. Get one that is full-length and thicker than you think you might need. You'll sleep more comfortably and warmly. If you have an air mattress that is not self-inflating, invest in a small battery-operated air pump that fits your mattress.

- **PLAN FOR TASTY, FUN, AND EASY MEALS.** If you're not hiking to a backcountry campsite, there's no reason to skimp on food due to weight, so bring what you need. It's especially fun when camp-ing with others to cook and eat around the campfire. With a little planning, you can prepackage and precook some ingredients to make great meals with easy preparation and clean-up. You can find plenty of books and Web sites with suggestions: I like **www.freezerbagcooking.com.**

- **BRING A KID OR TWO.** I've taken lots of kids on camping, hiking, caving, canoeing, and fishing trips, and can testify that the outdoors seems all the more adventurous and wonderful when seen through the eyes of a fifth-grader spending his first night in a tent. Take your own kids, grandkids, nieces or nephews, of course, but how about also inviting a couple of their friends, a co-worker and his kids, or a friend and her daughter? The natural world can be transformational for kids, particu-larly in this era when video games and texting are replacing old-fashioned outdoor play. Pick your campground and activities appropriate to the age, experience, and energy level (usually high) of the kids. I've included several with interesting hikes, swimming beaches, interactive exhibits, and even kid-friendly programs. See also *Camping with Kids* by Goldie Gendler Silverman from Menasha Ridge Press for suggestions and safety considerations.

CAMPING ETIQUETTE

Here are some simple tips to keep you on good terms with your camping neighbors, camp-ground personnel, and all of us who will come camping after you.

OBTAIN ALL PERMITS AND AUTHORIZATIONS REQUIRED Make sure you check in, pay your fee, and mark your site as directed. If the sign says to check in first, but you'd like to visually scope out the sites first, just ask.

FOLLOW THE CAMPGROUND'S RULES Observe rules regarding building fires, facility usage, parking, check-out times, number of people per site, etc.; ask if you need an excep-tion. If the rule says six people per site, but your nephew makes seven, check in advance if that would be acceptable. Most campground hosts are flexible with reasonable requests.

LEAVE ONLY FOOTPRINTS Be sensitive to the ground beneath you. Be sure to place all garbage in designated receptacles or pack it out if none is available. If there was trash when you arrived, take care of it as well, and leave the campsite better than you found it. Never burn trash—trash smoke smells and trash debris in a fire ring is unsightly.

BE COURTEOUS TO OTHER CAMPERS, HIKERS, BIKERS, AND OTHERS YOU ENCOUNTER:

- Respect their privacy and space unless invited—don't hike through their site to get to yours.

- If there are other choices, don't set up camp next to someone who has obviously selected a secluded site. It may be the best area of the campground, but they got there first, so you look elsewhere.

- Avoid, if you can, arriving late at night and attempting to set up camp in the glare of your headlights. If you must arrive late, look for a site away from others, plan to light a lantern, unload all at once (so you don't have to keep slamming car doors), and set up quietly.

- Keep the noise level down in your party, even if it's not officially quiet hours.

- If you camp with a dog, be sure it doesn't bark at passersby or noises in the night. Keep it leashed and clean up after it. Dog waste is not the same as wild animal waste. Those camping after you won't want to deal with it, and it can be harmful to the environment.

PLAN AHEAD Know your equipment, your ability, and the area in which you are camping, and prepare accordingly. Be self-sufficient at all times; carry necessary supplies for changes in weather and other conditions.

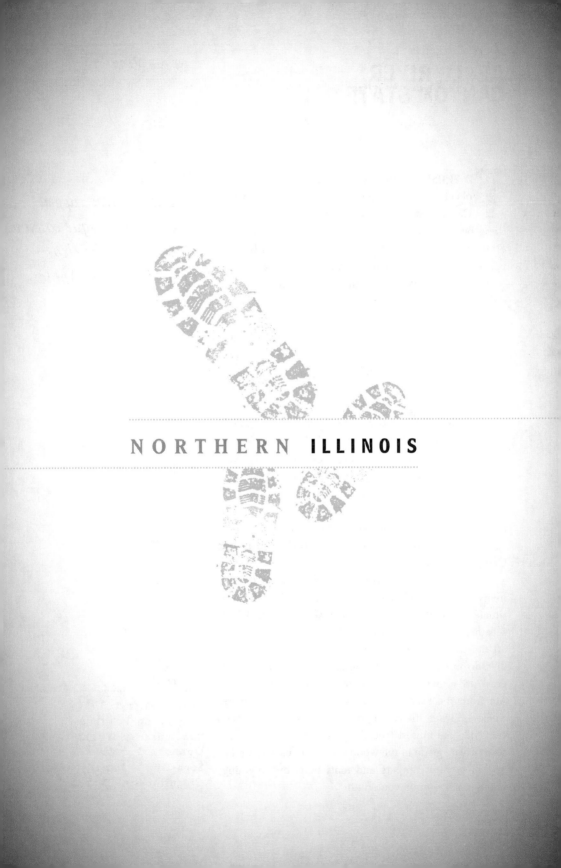

NORTHERN ILLINOIS

1
APPLE RIVER
CANYON STATE PARK

TO THOSE OF US FROM THE FLAT FARMLANDS of central Illinois, the topography of Apple River Canyon State Park is a pleasant surprise—can these bluffs and ravines really be part of the Prairie State? Amazingly, yes—this northwest corner of Illinois is something of a geologic island, having escaped the scouring of Ice Age glaciers that leveled hills and filled valleys elsewhere in the state. The same glaciers also blocked the Apple River's outlet, forcing it to carve a new channel southwest. The result is a rugged and picturesque canyon, with towering dolomite cliffs overlooking the clear, bubbling waters of the river below.

The campground, too, is a nice surprise, offering more peace and privacy than I usually expect from drive-in sites at a state park. There are few amenities— no concession or showers, and only a single electric site—but that keeps away the big RVs, and the regulars who camp here year after year are fine with that.

As you enter Apple River Canyon from the east on Canyon Road, pass Walnut Grove youth campground and the park office on the left. At the T-intersection, turn right and head uphill to the entrance to Canyon Ridge Campground on the left.

The layout of Canyon Ridge is similar to that of many state park campgrounds—two loops, with sites situated around the outside and inside of each. What sets this campground apart are the trees: many of these 50 sites are beautifully secluded from one another by the surrounding woods. Some are accessed by a short grass drive that angles back so you can't even see the site from the road. Even on an average non-holiday weekend, when the campground may be 50 to 75 percent full, you almost feel like you're camping at your own private glade in the woods. You will usually find a mix of pop-up campers and tents here, but anything much larger simply wouldn't fit.

> *Explore this rugged and picturesque canyon carved by the clear waters of the Apple River.*

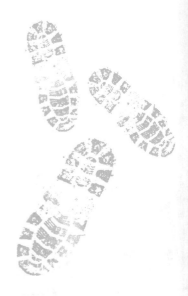

RATINGS

Beauty: ✿ ✿ ✿ ✿ ✿
Privacy: ✿ ✿ ✿ ✿
Spaciousness: ✿ ✿ ✿
Quiet: ✿ ✿ ✿ ✿
Security: ✿ ✿ ✿ ✿
Cleanliness: ✿ ✿ ✿ ✿ ✿

ADDRESS:	8763 East Canyon Road Apple River, IL 61001
OPERATED BY:	IDNR
CONTACT:	(815) 745-3302, www.dnr.state.il .us/lands/land mgt/parks/r1/ apple.htm
OPEN:	Year-round (Canyon Ridge Campground: Apr. 15–Oct. 31, Walnut Grove Campground: Nov. 1–Apr. 14)
SITES:	Class B: 1; Class C: 49
EACH SITE:	Picnic table, fire ring and grate; electric (Class B only)
ASSIGNMENT:	First come, first served
REGISTRATION:	Register at the office first
FACILITIES:	Water spigots, vault toilets
PARKING:	At site
FEE:	Class B: $18 per night, Class C: $8 per night
ELEVATION:	847 feet
RESTRICTIONS:	*Pets:* On leash only *Fires:* In fire rings only *Alcohol:* Not permitted *Vehicles:* 2 per site *Other:* 14-day limit; 1 RV and 1 tent, or 2 tents per site; 4 adults or 1 family per site; no swimming or boating

In the first loop, containing sites 1 through 23, I really like sites 2, 3, 8, 10, 11, and 15 for space, shade, and seclusion. Sites 1, 13, and 20 are also good choices, though with less shade. A few others, like 5, 6, and 16 through 19, are more open and close to the road, so not as private. Note that site 21 in this loop, originally intended for a campground host, is the only one with an electric hookup.

The second loop contains sites 24 through 50; those on the outside of the loop tend to be larger, better shaded, and farther from the road. Here the prize sites are 30 and 50. If you need two adjoining sites, 34 and 36 are a nice combination, with a short trail linking them. Whatever site you pick, head back to the office to register.

From November 1 to April 15, Canyon Ridge Campground is closed, so winter campers have to use Walnut Grove Campground, otherwise reserved for organized youth groups during the regular camping season. These 15 or so sites aren't nearly as private as those in the main campground, but during the off-season you'll have few, if any, neighbors here. The campground consists of a single half-circle drive, with parking in the middle. I'd pick a site at the back, away from the road, either to the right as you enter (west) or, even farther back, off the lane to the left (east). Note that the water is shut off during the winter, but there are vault toilets in the middle of the campground.

Hikers can explore the canyon via five excellent trails; some are rugged but well worth the effort to ascend to impressive overlooks. Others take you alongside the clear waters of the Apple River. All of them are 1 mile or less in length and start near the main parking and picnic area south of the campground, just across the river. Pine Ridge, Tower Rock, and River Route trails are more challenging, while Sunset and Primrose trails are easier hikes.

If you want more extensive hiking, head 35 miles or so southwest to the Mississippi River and Mississippi Palisades State Park. This very popular park features 15 miles of hiking trails. The trails in the southern part of the park are steep and rugged in places, leading to some spectacular views of the Mississippi River from

MAP

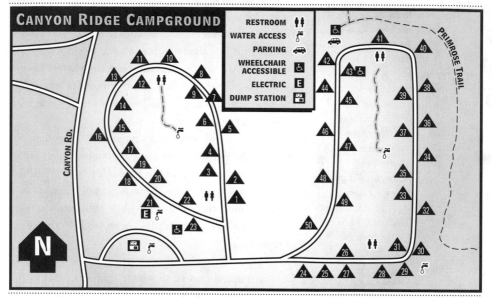

CANYON RIDGE CAMPGROUND

RESTROOM	
WATER ACCESS	
PARKING	
WHEELCHAIR ACCESSIBLE	
ELECTRIC	E
DUMP STATION	

CANYON RD.

PRIMROSE TRAIL

N

MAP

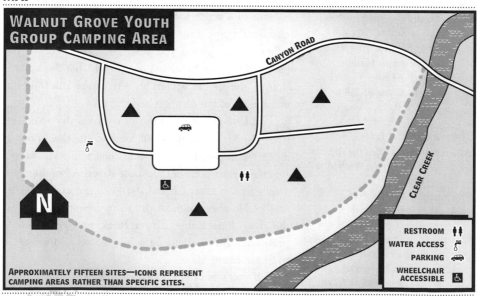

WALNUT GROVE YOUTH GROUP CAMPING AREA

CANYON ROAD

CLEAR CREEK

N

RESTROOM	
WATER ACCESS	
PARKING	
WHEELCHAIR ACCESSIBLE	

APPROXIMATELY FIFTEEN SITES—ICONS REPRESENT CAMPING AREAS RATHER THAN SPECIFIC SITES.

the limestone bluffs. Camping is also available, but the large campground is usually full of RVs—I'd rather stay elsewhere, and make this a day trip. This is also one of the few state parks in Illinois where rock climbing and rappelling are permitted—check with the park office for details. To get there from Apple River Canyon, go south from the campground 6.5 miles to US 20. Turn right (west) and go 20 miles to IL 84. Make a left (south) and go 15.3 miles to the north park entrance, on the left. Even if you don't want to hike, the drive along the Mississippi and to the overlooks in the park is well worth it.

GETTING THERE

From Rockford, take US 20 west about 45 miles to IL 78. Turn right (north) and go 6 miles to Canyon Road. Turn left and drive 3.5 miles to the park entrance.

GPS COORDINATES

UTM Zone 15T
Easting 0742552
Northing 4703831
Latitude N 42° 26' 55.9357"
Longitude W 90° 3' 1.9791"

2
LAKE LE-AQUA-NA
STATE PARK

DESPITE ITS SOUND, the name "Lake Le-Aqua-Na" does not come from some Native American language. It's actually the winning entry from a contest to name the lake, sponsored by the local sportsman's club in 1956: *aqua,* Latin for "water," stuck in the middle of the name of the nearby town of Lena.

While the name may be a bit unusual, it does reflect the pride that the staff and the local community take in this beautiful park. The 40-acre lake is the centerpiece, and everything around it is well maintained and clean, from the restrooms to the trails and even the campsite fire rings. It's busy on weekends but well worth a visit if you're looking for a comfortable place to camp, relax, and perhaps fish or swim.

Lake Le-Aqua-Na has two campgrounds, and both offer good choices for tent campers. As you enter the park, go straight; soon after the concession you'll come to the first campground, Pine Ridge, on the right. Its 25 sites are used almost exclusively by tent campers—you'll rarely find even a pop-up camper. Each site has a table and a big concrete fire ring.

Most sites are spacious, with more shade and privacy along the outside of the loop, sites 1 through 13. I like sites 5, 7, and 8 because they're a bit farther back from the road. Site 3 is also good—and near the toilets and water, if that's important. Sites 1 and 2 are a bit close to one another, but if you need two adjoining sites the combination is great because there is plenty of space and trees around. If you don't mind driving to use the showers in Hickory Hill Campground, Pine Ridge is smaller, usually less busy, and just a short walk from the lake and concession.

The only downside of Pine Ridge is that sites 20 through 24 are the youth group area and are occupied almost every weekend. Before you panic and imagine camping next to a Boy Scout Jamboree, however, note

> *Lake Le-Aqua-Na is busy on weekends but is a comfortable place to camp, relax, fish, and swim.*

RATINGS

Beauty: ✿ ✿ ✿ ✿
Privacy: ✿ ✿ ✿
Spaciousness: ✿ ✿ ✿
Quiet: ✿ ✿ ✿ ✿
Security: ✿ ✿ ✿ ✿
Cleanliness: ✿ ✿ ✿ ✿ ✿

ADDRESS:	8542 North Lake Road, Lena, IL
OPERATED BY:	IDNR
CONTACT:	(815) 369-4282, www.dnr.state .il.us/lands//land mgt/parks/r1/ leaquana.htm
OPEN:	Year-round
SITES:	At Pine Ridge, 24 Class B and 1 Class A; at Hickory Hill, 11 Class B and 142 Class A
EACH SITE:	Electric at Class A only; picnic table and fire ring
ASSIGNMENT:	First come, first served; sites 16–43 at Hickory Hill are reservable May 1–Oct. 31
REGISTRATION:	Set up, then park staff will come by
FACILITIES:	Water spigots, vault toilets; shower house (no water Nov.–Apr.)
PARKING:	At site
FEE:	Class A: $20 per night, $30 per night holidays; Class B: $10 per night; all sites $2 less when showers are closed; $5 reservation fee
ELEVATION:	926 feet
RESTRICTIONS:	*Pets:* On leash only *Fires:* In fire rings only *Alcohol:* Not permitted *Vehicles:* 2 per site *Other:* 14-day limit; 1 RV and 1 tent, or 2 tents per site; 4 adults or 1 family per site

that the area is small, and so are most groups that use it. They usually reserve well in advance, so you can call ahead to see if a youth group is expected and how large it might be.

Cross the road from Pine Ridge and walk down the hill to the lake. Follow the trail left along the shore, and you'll come to a secluded bench where you can fish or just sit and enjoy the view—the sunrise is nice from here. Continue around the bend to reach the small snack bar, where you can stop in for a cup of coffee and breakfast or lunch. While you're there, take a look at the fishing photos along the wall and in the albums. You can also rent canoes, pedal boats, or rowboats, and pick up limited camping or fishing supplies at the snack bar. Let them know if you need ice or firewood, and they'll deliver it to your campsite at specified times. New concessionaires took over mid-season in 2008, and in 2009 they plan to offer a more extensive menu, including weekend dinner specials. They're open daily May 1 to September 30 from 7 a.m.

Farther down the road from Pine Ridge is Hickory Hill Campground. All but 11 of these 153 sites have electrical hookups, so this is RV territory. However, if you are lucky enough to snag one, the four non-electric tent sites on the left as you drive in are great. Each is situated well back in the surrounding woods, but you can drive on the grass right to your site. Sites 151 and 152 are particularly private, nestled in a grove of trees but within a short walk of the shower building.

The other seven non-electric sites are 1 through 7, located on a hilltop to the right as you enter the campground. These are fairly spacious but wide open with little shade. If you want electricity, you'll probably find a bit more privacy and shade at the back, around sites 86 and 87. You can expect this campground to be busy on an average weekend. If the campground hosts at Hickory Hill are the same enthusiastic couple I met in 2008 (and they're planning to return), it's well worth stopping to visit with them. She'll have a stack of brochures on both the park and surrounding attractions. He's the fisherman and will be glad to tell you what's biting and how to catch it.

MAP

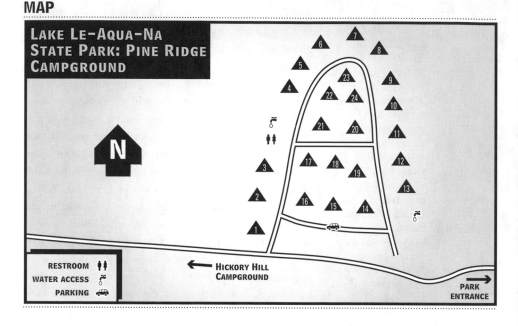

LAKE LE-AQUA-NA
STATE PARK: PINE RIDGE
CAMPGROUND

N

RESTROOM	👥
WATER ACCESS	🚰
PARKING	🚗

← HICKORY HILL
CAMPGROUND

PARK
ENTRANCE

Fishing is popular at Lake Le-Aqua-Na. In addition to containing typical Illinois species like crappie, bluegill, channel catfish, and largemouth bass, the lake is just far enough north to accommodate northern pike. When I was there the campground host had just recently caught a 30-inch pike.

Kids will enjoy the small, free swimming beach near the park entrance, and adults will at least find it a good place to cool off. If you want chlorinated swimming, check out Splash Land water park in Lena, which has a couple of pools and an awesome water slide. A coupon from the park will get you a discount. Call (815) 369-9165 for more information.

GETTING THERE

From Rockford, take US 20 west about 40 miles to IL 73. Turn right (north) and drive 1.7 miles into Lena. Turn left on Lena Street, and go 0.4 miles to Freedom Street. Turn right and head 3 miles north to the park entrance, on the left.

GPS COORDINATES

UTM Zone 16T
Easting 0267646
Northing 4700350
Latitude N 42° 25' 14.4542"
Longitude W 89° 49' 27.0729"

3
SUGAR RIVER
FOREST PRESERVE

> *Camp, hike, or canoe along the serene and isolated banks of the lazy Sugar River.*

ONE OF THE MOST SERENE and isolated rivers in northern Illinois is the Sugar, which meanders lazily from Wisconsin south toward Rockford. Its waters are clear, flowing over sandy soil, along low banks, and by sandy bluffs. The surrounding countryside is mostly unspoiled by development, thanks largely to Winnebago County, which has set aside 529 acres along its banks to form the Sugar River Forest Preserve. Sugar River's campground is popular, but there are also good spots for tent camping along the river.

As you enter on Forest Preserve Road, take the right fork toward the campground. Pine Tree campground has 70 electric sites, situated around a single loop within a large grove of pines, as the name suggests. The sites aren't secluded, but they are spacious, compared to those at most park RV campgrounds, in addition to being flat and fairly well shaded. The sites around the outside of the loop (sites 32 through 70) are deeper and roomier, and there are more trees toward the back—site 46 is the best here. This campground is about half to three-quarters full most non-holiday weekends.

Much more secluded and spacious, but less shaded, are the 12 walk-in sites along the Sugar River. Go left at the campground entrance, and you'll to come the small parking area, with vault toilets and a water spigot. From here it's an easy, flat walk of about 400 to 800 feet to any of the sites, and you can bring a wagon to haul your gear, if you want. This area is also popular—about three-quarters full most weekends.

Walk east from the parking lot to site 10 on the river—sites 4 through 9 are to the left, 11 and 12 to the right, and 1 through 3 are away from the river, accessed by short trail from site 7. These are all situated on sandy, grass-covered soil, with no brush or trees between them. Each has a table and a fire ring, and sites 4 through 12 are just a few steps from the riverbank. On the left, I

RATINGS

Beauty: ✿ ✿ ✿ ✿
Privacy: ✿ ✿ ✿
Spaciousness: ✿ ✿ ✿ ✿ ✿
Quiet: ✿ ✿ ✿ ✿
Security: ✿ ✿ ✿ ✿
Cleanliness: ✿ ✿ ✿ ✿

like site 4 because it's at the end of the row, so neighbors won't be walking by to get to their sites, and it has some trees around. Site 1 is more secluded and wooded, though not on the river. Site 6 also has some shade.

Farthest from the other sites is the combination of sites 11 and 12, which afford lots of room to spread out. Since the forest preserve allows up to three tents per site, these would be ideal for a small group. Wherever you choose, set up and staff will come by to register you. Unfortunately, walk-in camping fees do not include use of the shower house in the main campground.

Because of their location, these sites may flood in the early spring. Also, when I was there in August of 2008, the mosquitoes were terrible, even in the middle of the day. However, staff said there'd been a lot of flooding recently, and consequently they were much worse than usual. If you're hoping to come in the spring to mid-summer, call first for conditions and bring bug spray.

The best way to see the river is by canoe, and there are numerous access points along its length, from Wisconsin down to where it joins with the muddier but equally scenic Pecatonica. Note that the river is sometimes too high or low to canoe safely and tricky to navigate because of deadfall. However, as of 2008 there are no outfitters serving the Sugar in Illinois, so if you don't have your own canoe and means of shuttling, you'll have to be content exploring on foot. Sugar River Forest Preserve offers 6 miles of hiking trails, and Colored Sands Forest Preserve, to the north across Yale Road, adds another 2-mile loop. The latter is so named because of the unique 40-foot multicolored sandy bluff on the east bank, near a bend in the river. The hike from the entrance to the bluff is about 0.75 miles. To get there from Sugar River, go east on Yale Road to Hauley Road, turn left, continue 0.5 miles north to Haas Road, turn left again, and go 1 mile to the forest preserve entrance, on the left. Excellent trail maps for all the county forest preserves can be found on the district Web site, **www.wcfpd.org.**

Colored Sands is also home to the Sand Bluff Bird Observatory, which offers visitors a rare opportunity to participate in banding migrating birds. On spring and

KEY INFORMATION

ADDRESS: 10127 Forest Preserve Road, Durand, IL 61024

OPERATED BY: Winnebago County Forest Preserve District

CONTACT: (815) 629-2468, www.wcfpd.org/ preserves/sugar river.cfm

OPEN: Mid-April to mid-November

SITES: 12 walk-in sites and 70 vehicle-access sites

EACH SITE: Picnic table, fire ring; electric in main campground only

ASSIGNMENT: First come, first served

REGISTRATION: Set up and park personnel will come by

FACILITIES: Water spigots, vault toilets; shower house in main campground only

PARKING: At campsite or in lot

FEE: walk-in sites: $10 per night, electric sites: $17 per night

ELEVATION: 807 feet

RESTRICTIONS: *Pets:* On leash only *Fires:* In fire rings only *Alcohol:* Permitted *Vehicles:* 2 per site *Other:* 14-day limit; 3 tents per site; set up and register by 10 p.m.; no gathering of downed wood

MAP

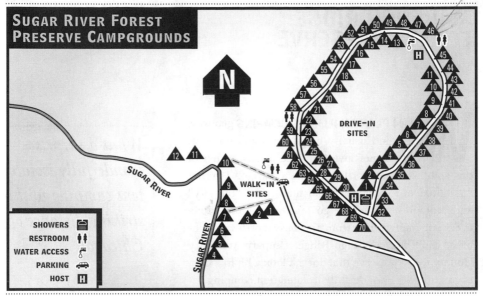

SUGAR RIVER FOREST PRESERVE CAMPGROUNDS

DRIVE-IN SITES

WALK-IN SITES

SHOWERS
RESTROOM
WATER ACCESS
PARKING
HOST

GETTING THERE

From I-39, take Exit 3 and head west on Rockton Road (CR 9) 8 miles to Forest Preserve Road. Turn right and drive 4.5 miles to the Sugar River Forest Preserve entrance.

GPS COORDINATES

UTM Zone 16T
Easting 0316187
Northing 4703648
Latitude N 42° 27' 48.1503"
Longitude W 89° 14' 8.6569"

fall weekends, volunteers use large mesh nets to trap birds, then gently measure their wingspans and attach an aluminum band to the leg, allowing their travels to be monitored. Over the years, they have banded more than 85,000 birds of 150-plus species. Large maps with pins indicate where those birds were later spotted throughout the Americas. Visitors are welcome and can help release birds. Banding takes place from March through May, and late August through November, and the annual Birdfest on Mother's Day weekend includes special activities for kids, raptor demonstrations, special exhibits, and food vendors. Call the forest preserve for more information, or check **www.birdfreak.com/winnebago-birding/colored-sands-forest-preserve.**

4

MARENGO RIDGE FOREST PRESERVE

WHEN I PLAN AN ILLINOIS CAMPING getaway, my mind usually gravitates south—or east, west, or northwest—in fact, to any corner of the state but the northeast, aka Chicago. I'm not enamored of expressways and malls, and "big city" and "camping" just don't go together for me. However, not many miles from the busy northwest suburbs, you'll find Marengo Ridge, a superb McHenry County forest preserve that doesn't look a bit like Chicago and offers wonderfully isolated tent camping.

As you enter the forest preserve off IL 23, head straight back to the Thomas Woods campground entrance and stop first at the trailer to register. Here you'll also find trail maps and can purchase firewood and ice. This southern loop of the campground has 18 sites especially for RVs, though only two, sites 0 and 4, have electric hookups. Tent campers can also use these sites.

Drive past RV sites 1 through 3 and turn left to enter the tent-only area with its 29 beautifully wooded sites. All of these sites have a table, fire ring with grill, and a flat, raised tent pad bordered by landscaping timbers and filled with fine crushed gravel. (You're not required to pitch your tent on the pad, however.) Most are well shaded under a mix of pine and hardwoods. You can pull into 7 of the sites, but far better for privacy are any of the 22 walk-in sites, which have been carefully laid out in separate sections of just a few sites each. The result is that even on busy weekends the campground doesn't feel crowded, and at many sites you'll find yourself nicely secluded from neighbors by the surrounding trees and brush.

You'll first pass sites 18 through 27 along the lower road. These are older and not quite as spread out as those on the ridge above, but there are still some excellent options here. In the first set of walk-ins, site 18 is the farthest from the others, though it is

> *What a surprise—wonderfully isolated tent camping within striking distance of Chicago!*

RATINGS

Beauty: ✩ ✩ ✩ ✩
Privacy: ✩ ✩ ✩ ✩ ✩
Spaciousness: ✩ ✩ ✩
Quiet: ✩ ✩ ✩ ✩
Security: ✩ ✩ ✩ ✩ ✩
Cleanliness: ✩ ✩ ✩ ✩ ✩

ADDRESS:	2411 South Route 23, Marengo, IL
OPERATED BY:	McHenry County Conservation District
CONTACT:	(815) 338-6223, www.mccdistrict.org/web/re-camping.htm
OPEN:	May 1–October 31
SITES:	29 tent sites (22 walk-in); 18 RV sites (2 electric)
EACH SITE:	Picnic table, fire ring
ASSIGNMENT:	First come, first served; reservations available by phone
REGISTRATION:	At check-in trailer
FACILITIES:	Water spigots, vault toilets
PARKING:	At site; at lot for walk-in sites
FEE:	$8 per tent per night non-electric ($12 out of county residents); $16 per tent per night electric ($24 out-of-county residents)
ELEVATION:	893 feet
RESTRICTIONS:	*Pets:* On leash only *Fires:* In fire rings only *Alcohol:* Not within 100 feet of a parking area *Vehicles:* 1 per site (tent area) *Other:* Check-in by 7 p.m.; no amplified music; 3-day maximum stay (2-day extension possible); 8 people per site except for larger families

also right along a hiking trail. Site 21 is also in a pretty spot by itself.

Turn right past site 27 and head uphill to the newer tent sites. Most of the walk-in sites here are well separated from one another, with just enough distance between you and the parking lot so you're not disturbed by vehicle lights and noises. The best are those farthest from their respective parking areas: sites 29, 30, 34, 36, 44, and 46. If you and a friend need a pair of sites, 36 and 37 are adjoining, linked by a short trail. My favorite is 44, all by itself down a short trail, about 150 feet from parking, and well worth the walk. If you prefer a pull-in site, 39, 40, and 42 are good choices.

With its proximity to Chicago, Marengo Ridge is popular, particularly on weekends, so it's wise to reserve your site in advance by phone. There's no additional charge, but weekend reservations must be made by noon on the Thursday prior.

The terrain around Marengo Ridge can best be described as undulating, the result of successive waves of glaciers that deposited mounds of sand and gravel as they melted and receded. The forest preserve itself rests atop part of the Marengo Moraine, a ridge that marks the westernmost limits of the Wisconsin ice sheet and stretches from the state line south about 40 miles. The resulting panorama can best be appreciated from the observation area south of the preserve entrance, where you can look out for miles over the rolling prairie. Look for the interpretive sign that describes what you're seeing and puts it all in geologic perspective.

You can further explore Marengo Ridge through the 5-mile network of hiking trails. The southern loop descends into the valley from the observation point, and the northern loops wind through a mix of pine, oak, and hickory forest, up and down the hills, and past intermittent streams.

If Marengo Ridge is the best place to tent camp in McHenry County, Moraine Hills State Park is a prime choice for hiking and biking. This 2,200-acre park east of Marengo is also characterized by glacially formed topography—rolling hills, marshes, bogs, and 48-acre Lake Defiance, one of the few glacial lakes in Illinois that has remained largely undeveloped. Over 10 miles

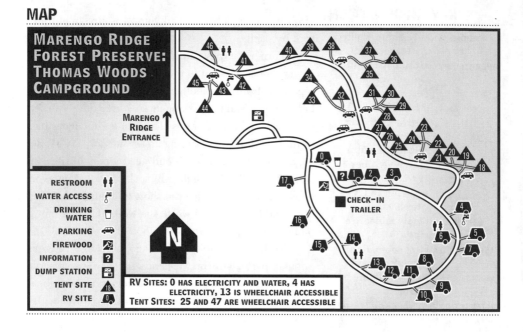

MARENGO RIDGE FOREST PRESERVE: THOMAS WOODS CAMPGROUND

MARENGO RIDGE ENTRANCE

RESTROOM	👫
WATER ACCESS	🚰
DRINKING WATER	🥤
PARKING	🚗
FIREWOOD	🪵
INFORMATION	?
DUMP STATION	
TENT SITE	▲18
RV SITE	🚐0

CHECK-IN TRAILER

N

RV SITES: 0 HAS ELECTRICITY AND WATER, 4 HAS ELECTRICITY, 13 IS WHEELCHAIR ACCESSIBLE
TENT SITES: 25 AND 47 ARE WHEELCHAIR ACCESSIBLE

of well-maintained trails traverse the park in four connected loops, all paved or surfaced with crushed limestone, and very popular with cyclists. Whether on bike or foot, keep an eye out for the incredible diversity of plant and animal life present, including one of Illinois' largest colonies of rare carnivorous pitcher plants.

You can also fish along the Fox River or from the boardwalk at Lake Defiance, and boat rental and snacks are available at the concession from April through October. To get there from Marengo Ridge, go 2 miles south on IL 23 to IL 176 (Telegraph Street) in Marengo. Turn left, proceed 22 miles east, over the Fox River, and turn left onto River Road. The park entrance is 2 miles north. Call (815) 385-1624 or check **www.dnr.state.il.us/lands/ landmgt/parks/r2/morhills.htm** for more information.

GETTING THERE

From Interstate 90 (Northwest Tollway), take Exit 36 and go 9 miles north on US 20 to Marengo. Turn right onto IL 23 (State Street). Go 2.5 miles north to forest preserve entrance on the right.

GPS COORDINATES

UTM Zone 16T
Easting 0367504
Northing 4682555
Latitude N 42° 17' 2.2521"
Longitude W 88° 36' 25.1807"

LOUD THUNDER
FOREST PRESERVE

LakeGe orge, nestled amid the surrounding forested hills, is a tranquil spot for canoeing, hiking, and camping.

RATINGS

Beauty: ✪ ✪ ✪ ✪
Privacy: ✪ ✪ ✪
Spaciousness: ✪ ✪ ✪
Quiet: ✪ ✪ ✪ ✪
Security: ✪ ✪ ✪ ✪ ✪
Cleanliness: ✪ ✪ ✪ ✪ ✪

AT 1,621 ACRES, LOUD THUNDER is the largest and most picturesque of the Rock Island County Forest Preserves. There are miles of multiuse trails, beautiful views of the Mississippi River, and 167-acre Lake George, nestled amid the forested hills. With the Quad Cities just to the north, Loud Thunder is popular on weekends, but five separate campgrounds with a total of 115 sites offer plenty of choices for tent campers.

The first campground you'll see as you enter Loud Thunder is Silva, 0.6 miles from Interstate 92 on the left. Silva offers 19 sites located along a ridge stretching toward Lake George. A bit of brush separates the sites from one another. Those on the right as you enter (west) overlook a small valley, while those on the east have trees behind them. Sites 47 and 48 at the end are a bit more spacious and set back from the road, as are sites 39 through 43 on the east.

The entrance to the Riverview Campground loop is 0.25 miles past Silva on the right, then 0.3 miles down the hill to the Mississippi River. There's not much shade or privacy, but 11 of these 34 sites (24 through 34) offer impressive vistas right at the riverside. You're actually not even looking across the entire width of the Mississippi here, only about 0.25 miles to Andalusia Island in the middle of the river. The sites at the eastern edge (33 and 34) are a bit farther from traffic, but this campground is still the most popular nonelectric one at Loud Thunder, so don't count on solitude most weekends.

Head down the hill from the Riverview entrance, across the dam, and turn left at the park office. The left fork leads to the boat ramp and concession, the right to White Oak, Indian Meadows, and Horse Corral campgrounds. White Oak has 26 electric sites for RVs only, no tents allowed. Adjacent Indian Meadows has 22 sites ranged along a ridge with some brush and trees between them. Sites 42 and 44 on the east (as you enter) are a bit larger and overlook the lake below. The sites around the loop at the end of the road are too close, with the exception of 37, which has more surrounding trees.

At the end of the road, Horse Corral is the least used of the campgrounds, and fortunately its 14 numbered sites are open to all campers, not just equestrians. Most sites here are close to the road and in an open field with little shade. To the left, however, sites 51 and 52 are more private, set back some distance. And to reach the two most secluded sites in all of Loud Thunder (my favorites), turn right onto the gravel road as you enter the campground and continue about 600 feet along the edge of the field. You'll come to sites 61 and 62, situated all by themselves in a wooded opening. If you didn't have a campground map (or this book), you wouldn't even know they existed.

Each campground at Loud Thunder has toilets and at least one water spigot. All campers can use the excellent shower house outside White Oak.

Loud Thunder offers hikers, mountain bikers, and equestrians diverse opportunities to explore the forested ridges surrounding Lake George and the bottomlands along the Mississippi. The trails north of Loud Thunder Road are limited to foot traffic, while most of those to the south are designated for multiuse. For an easier hike with wonderful views of the river, head east from Riverview Campground on the east branch of Hauberg Trail. You can hike the entire 1.2 miles to the parking lot on I-92, then return via part of the Sac-Fox Trail. More challenging is the southern portion of Sac-Fox, about 8 miles total, including a 4.6-mile loop that begins at Horse Corral Campground. This section is popular with mountain bikers as well. For detailed trail maps, check the excellent and informative Forest Preserve District website: **www.ricfpd.org.**

Fishing and boating are popular at Loud Thunder, both on Lake George and the Mississippi. Since boats on the lake are limited to trolling motors, it's quiet, too, and a tranquil spot for canoeing. Lyle's Landing (the lakeside concession) rents canoes, kayaks, paddleboats, hydro bikes, and johnboats and sells bait, tackle, and snacks. Call (309) 795-1070 for more information.

KEY INFORMATION

ADDRESS:	19408 Loud Thunder Road, Illinois City, IL 61259
OPERATED BY:	Rock Island County Conservation District
CONTACT:	(309) 795-1040, www.ricfpd.org/ RICFPD/ LoudThunder .aspx?id=9790
OPEN:	Apr. 1–Oct. 31
SITES:	White Oak Campground (electric and water hookups): 26 sites; other campgrounds (nonelectric): 89 sites
EACH SITE:	Picnic table, fire ring
ASSIGNMENT:	First come, first served
REGISTRATION:	Set up, then ranger collects fees at night
FACILITIES:	Water spigots, vault and flush toilets, shower house
PARKING:	At site
FEE:	White Oak Campground: $14 per night; other campgrounds: $11 per night ($1 less for county residents, $2 less for senior citizens)
ELEVATION:	722 feet
RESTRICTIONS:	*Pets:* On leash only *Fires:* In fire rings only *Alcohol:* Permitted *Vehicles:* 2 per site *Other:* 14-day limit; 1 RV or 1 tent per site

MAP

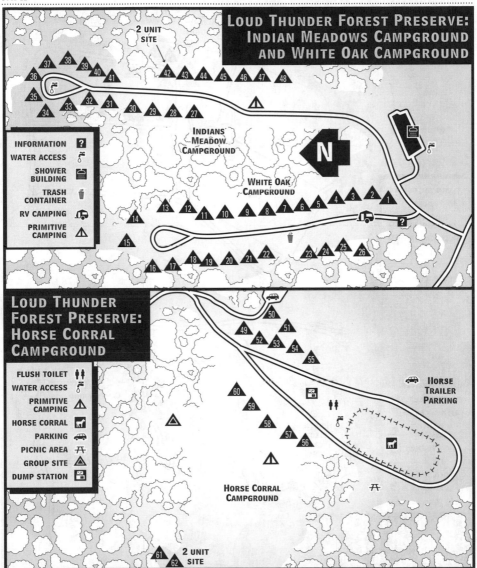

LOUD THUNDER FOREST PRESERVE: INDIAN MEADOWS CAMPGROUND AND WHITE OAK CAMPGROUND

2 UNIT SITE

INDIANS' MEADOW CAMPGROUND

WHITE OAK CAMPGROUND

INFORMATION	
WATER ACCESS	
SHOWER BUILDING	
TRASH CONTAINER	
RV CAMPING	
PRIMITIVE CAMPING	

LOUD THUNDER FOREST PRESERVE: HORSE CORRAL CAMPGROUND

FLUSH TOILET	
WATER ACCESS	
PRIMITIVE CAMPING	
HORSE CORRAL	
PARKING	
PICNIC AREA	
GROUP SITE	
DUMP STATION	

HORSE TRAILER PARKING

HORSE CORRAL CAMPGROUND

2 UNIT SITE

Loud Thunder is named after the son of Sauk Indian leader Black Hawk, whose people occupied the area from about 1750 to 1831, when they were forced across the Mississippi by encroaching settlement. His courageous but ill-fated war in 1832 to reclaim his home village eventually made him a local hero. Black Hawk State Historic Site on Rock Island provides a fascinating overview of his life and the culture of the Sauk and Fox tribes. The site was closed in late 2008 due to budget cuts, but I expect it to reopen in 2009. Check **www.blackhawk park.org** for current information.

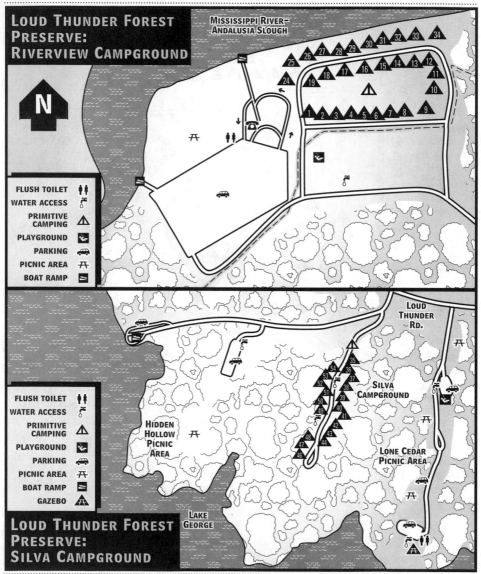

LOUD THUNDER FOREST PRESERVE: RIVERVIEW CAMPGROUND

MISSISSIPPI RIVER–ANDALUSIA SLOUGH

FLUSH TOILET
WATER ACCESS
PRIMITIVE CAMPING
PLAYGROUND
PARKING
PICNIC AREA
BOAT RAMP

FLUSH TOILET
WATER ACCESS
PRIMITIVE CAMPING
PLAYGROUND
PARKING
PICNIC AREA
BOAT RAMP
GAZEBO

LOUD THUNDER RD.

SILVA CAMPGROUND

HIDDEN HOLLOW PICNIC AREA

LONE CEDAR PICNIC AREA

LAKE GEORGE

LOUD THUNDER FOREST PRESERVE: SILVA CAMPGROUND

GETTING THERE

From Interstate 280, take Exit 11 onto IL 92 W toward Andalusia. Drive 1.5 miles south and turn right, following IL 92. Go 12 miles west through Andalusia to Loud Thunder Road and turn right into the forest preserve.

GPS COORDINATES

UTM Zone 15T

Easting 0682078

Northing 4588991

Latitude N 41° 25' 54.6946"

Longitude W 90° 49' 14.8704"

6

JOHNSON–SAUK TRAIL STATE RECREATION AREA

> *Camp under the tall pines, and enjoy some of the extra conveniences Johnson–Sauk Trail offers.*

MORE THAN THREE HUNDRED YEARS AGO, the Sauk, among other Native American tribes, traveled through north-central Illinois on their way from Lake Michigan to the confluence of the Rock and Mississippi Rivers. Today's travelers coming to the Johnson–Sauk Trail State Park can enjoy the same rolling terrain, along with a scenic lake and some nice conveniences to make their stay a bit more comfortable.

As you enter the park from IL 78, pass the distinctive round barn and take the next right into the Chief Keokuk Campground. You'll immediately be struck by the stately tall pines standing along the road and overshadowing these well-spaced campsites. Stop first at the small parking lot to the left, one of two that serve the 25 non-electric tent sites. Though these are technically walk-in sites, this campground boasts a gravel access lane between the parking lots. You can drive close to your site just for unloading or loading, and then park at either end. You get the best of both worlds—you don't have to carry your gear far, and vehicle noise is limited near the campsites.

All these sites are well shaded by the pines, and my favorites are toward the east end. Sites 97 and 98 are popular, offering plenty of space and a great view of the lake—you may need to arrive early on a weekend to get one of these. Just to the west, 96, 95, and 94 are also nice. Among the others, 78, 82, 83, 84, 87, 88, and 89 are all good choices, sufficiently spacious and set back from the gravel road. The remaining sites are less desirable, being too small, too close to the road, or too crowded with trees.

The 71 electric sites are situated south of the tent area. There's plenty of space between these, but the ones in the largest loop, sites 32 through 72, aren't as well shaded. If you want electricity, the better sites for

RATINGS

Beauty: ✿ ✿ ✿ ✿
Privacy: ✿ ✿ ✿
Spaciousness: ✿ ✿ ✿
Quiet: ✿ ✿ ✿ ✿
Security: ✿ ✿ ✿ ✿
Cleanliness: ✿ ✿ ✿ ✿ ✿

tents are along the road past the host. Site 5, 6, 8, or 9 would be my choice, each with plenty of space for setting up a couple of tents.

Whatever you choose, select your site, set up, and then register with the campground host at site 1 or 2, or with park staff, who will come around in the evening if no host is available. All campers can use the very clean, well-maintained shower house, which also includes separate, wheelchair-accessible men's and women's restrooms and showers—a bit of additional privacy not usually found at campgrounds. Note that all water in the campground is turned off from November through April.

The Lakeside Restaurant and store, east of the campground, will quickly spoil you. Large and attractive, the restaurant has a full menu and offers dinner specials such as fish and steak on Fridays. You can eat inside and enjoy the air-conditioning or dine outside at one of the canopied tables overlooking the lake—watch for the families of ground squirrels that the concessionaire feeds. You'll often find a crowd here on weekends, both campers and locals. And if you don't want to walk the short distance to the restaurant, they'll deliver for free—yes, right to your campsite! They have only three delivery times—10 a.m., 2 p.m., and 8 p.m.—so you may use this service more for firewood or ice than food, but it's nice to know about. The store carries food as well as camping and fishing supplies, and you can rent paddleboats, rowboats, canoes, or flat-bottomed boats with a trolling motor, even overnight if you're a registered camper. The concession's season is April 1 through October 1, open every day but Monday. Call them at (309) 852-5253 for details or to request delivery.

If you come on a weekend between May and October, visit Ryan's Round Barn. Constructed between 1908 and 1910 for a Dr. Ryan as part of his cattle farm, this unique building featured some innovative labor-saving systems for its time. It's been carefully restored by local volunteers, who open the barn for tours on selected Saturdays from 1 to 4 p.m. and are available to answer questions.

Johnson–Sauk Trail isn't a hiker's paradise, but if you want to work off the dinner you had at the Lakeside Restaurant, it does offer eight short (0.25-mile to

KEY INFORMATION

ADDRESS:	28616 Sauk Trail Rd., Kewanee, IL
OPERATED BY:	IDNR
CONTACT:	(309) 853-5589, www.dnr.state.il.us/lands/land mgt/parks/r1/johnson.htm
OPEN:	Year-round
SITES:	Class C: 25 walk-in tent sites; Class A: 71 electric sites
EACH SITE:	Electric only in Class A; picnic table, ground grill
ASSIGNMENT:	First come, first served
REGISTRATION:	Set up first, then register with campground host if available, or park staff will come by
FACILITIES:	Water spigots, vault toilets; shower house (no water Nov.–Apr.)
PARKING:	At site (Class A); in lot (Class C)
FEE:	Class A: $20 per night, $30 per night holidays; Class D: $8 per night; all $2 less when showers are closed
ELEVATION:	781 feet
RESTRICTIONS:	*Pets:* On leash only *Fires:* In fire rings only *Alcohol:* Permitted *Vehicles:* 2 per site *Other:* 14-day limit; 1 RV and 1 tent, or 2 tents per site; 4 adults or 1 family per site

MAP

JOHNSON–SAUK TRAIL STATE RECREATION AREA: CHIEF KEOKUK CAMPGROUND

SHOWER	
RESTROOM	
WATER ACCESS	
PARKING	
DUMP STATION	
DUMPSTER	

CAMPGROUND ENTRANCE

SAUK TRAIL RD.

N

GETTING THERE

From I-80, take Exit 33 onto IL 78 south toward Annawan. Drive 6 miles south, then turn left at the park entrance sign.

From Kewanee, go north on IL 78 (Main Street) 11.5 miles and turn right at the park entrance sign.

GPS COORDINATES

UTM Zone 16T
Easting 0256891
Northing 4578499
Latitude N 41° 19' 16.7586"
Longitude W 89° 54' 16.7343"

1-mile) well-maintained trails in the day-use area of the park. Cyclists who want more exercise can check out the historic Hennepin Canal Trail, which runs almost 105 miles along the restored canal towpath. You can connect with the trail at a number of places, but the closest is 6 miles north of Johnson–Sauk off IL 78, 0.3 miles past I-80. The canal is also an easy canoe route, but you do have to portage around the remaining non-functioning locks. For more information and a detailed map, visit the excellent visitor center, open Monday through Friday, 8 a.m. to 4 p.m. Call (815) 454-2328. To get there, go 12 miles east on I-80 to Exit 45, then head south 1 mile to the sign on the right.

7
CHANNAHON AND GEBHARD WOODS STATE PARKS

THE YEAR 1848 WITNESSED an economic development that would forever change Illinois and the whole Midwest—the opening of the Illinois & Michigan Canal. Dug entirely by hand, this 96-mile corridor linked Lake Michigan with the Illinois River, completing a water route from the eastern seaboard to the Gulf of Mexico. At the crossroads, Chicago would prosper as a major transportation hub.

Thanks to the efforts of many volunteers, today the historic canal continues to be good for business, now as a recreational venue for hikers, anglers, cyclists, canoeists, and campers. And of the several places to camp along the way, two of the best for tent campers are Channahon State Park and Gebhard Woods State Park.

Though not quite the northern end of the I & M Canal Trail, Channahon State Park is a good place to start the most scenic stretch. This small park has 19 unnumbered walk-in tent sites scattered in a field between the office and the canal, each with a picnic table and fire ring. The 14 sites in the area by the parking lot are all fairly close together, and it would feel crowded if they were all full. However, this little campground never fills up—a busy non-holiday weekend might see six tents. The closest sites are just a few steps from the parking lot. The five sites at the northern end are my favorites, though—they're about 500 feet from parking but offer more space, shade, and seclusion. Water and vault toilets are at this end of the grounds, and if there's firewood stacked by the end of the fence, you're welcome to use it.

About 15 miles southwest by road (or 15.1 miles down the I & M Canal Trail) is Gebhard Woods State Park. Here you have to walk 0.2 miles to get to the camping area. From the northwest end of the parking lot, walk about 800 feet east along what looks like a service lane, and turn left at the camping sign. The nine

> *Either park is a quiet base from which to hike, bike, or canoe the historic I & M Canal.*

RATINGS

Beauty: ✩ ✩ ✩
Privacy: ✩ ✩
Spaciousness: ✩ ✩ ✩ ✩
Quiet: ✩ ✩ ✩ ✩
Security: ✩ ✩ ✩ ✩
Cleanliness: ✩ ✩ ✩ ✩

unnumbered tent sites are spaced along the northern edge of a large open field bordered by Nettle Creek. Each is marked by a fire ring and table. Though there's plenty of space between sites, there's not much else, so no sense of privacy. Some are decently shaded—the best is the site in the middle by the creek. You'll find water and restrooms near the pavilion across the field.

At Gebhard Woods, as at Channahon, you probably won't have many camping neighbors. On a fair weather, non-holiday weekend, there may be just three sites taken. The only regular exceptions are the second weekend in June—an annual dulcimer festival—and one weekend in April when Boy Scouts camp here, which is always scheduled in advance, so call first if you're thinking of an April trip.

At either of these places you'll feel more like you're camping in a city park than in the wilderness—understandable, since both are surrounded by city. Of the two, I like Channahon better for camping. I think it's because you don't have to walk quite as far, yet the sites at the back of the campground seem more secluded and shaded than those at Gebhard Woods. Also, camping isolationist that I am, I enjoyed the fact that Channahon was completely empty, whereas Gebhard Woods had a few day visitors using the park during my stay.

Most come here for access to the I & M Canal Trail—61.5 miles of restored towpath, once the domain of the horses and mules that pulled the canal boats. It's an excellent flat and scenic trek for hikers but is especially popular with cyclists. The surface is crushed limestone and the gradient slight, so it's a relaxing hike or ride, with plenty of historic and natural sights, and restrooms and water access along the way. From Channahon, it's just 3 miles to McKinley Woods, which also features primitive camping and about 2.5 miles of hiking trails (visit **www.fpdwc.org** for a trail map).

Before you start out, be sure to get an I & M Canal Trail map, which should be available at the Channahon or Gebhard Woods offices. If you want to get one in advance, visit **www.dnr.state.il.us/lands/land mgt/parks/i&m/main.htm**. You'll also find the mileage chart at **www.bikelib.org/mapstrails/iandmmaps.htm**.

MAP

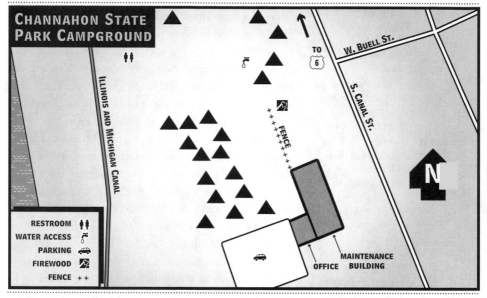

CHANNAHON STATE PARK CAMPGROUND

ILLINOIS AND MICHIGAN CANAL

TO 6

W. BUELL ST.

S. CANAL ST.

FENCE

N

OFFICE

MAINTENANCE BUILDING

RESTROOM	👬
WATER ACCESS	
PARKING	
FIREWOOD	
FENCE	+ +

MAP

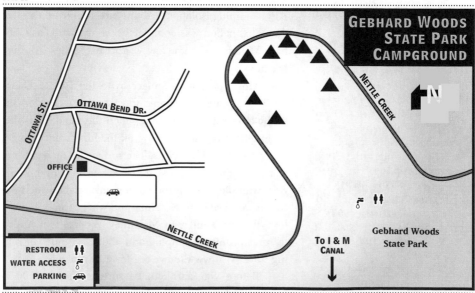

GEBHARD WOODS STATE PARK CAMPGROUND

OTTAWA ST.

OTTAWA BEND DR.

NETTLE CREEK

N

OFFICE

NETTLE CREEK

To I & M CANAL

Gebhard Woods State Park

RESTROOM	👬
WATER ACCESS	
PARKING	🚗

You can canoe portions of the canal, particularly the 15-mile stretch between Channahon and Gebhard Woods. Because there's little current, you can go in either direction. Unfortunately, there are currently no local outfitters, so you'll have to bring your own canoe if you want to experience the canal this way. Note that parts of this section sometimes become overgrown with vegetation during the summer, so call first to check on conditions.

To learn more about the fascinating history of the canal, check the Canal Corridor Association's Web site at **www.canalcor.org.** In June of 2008 they opened a visitor center in LaSalle that offers one-hour round-trip rides on an authentic replica of an original canal boat. Check **www.lasalleboat.org** for prices and schedules.

If you have time, Starved Rock and Mathiessen State Parks south of Utica are well worth visiting for the superb hiking through their deep, cool canyons. Starved Rock offers camping but is usually crowded. Mathiessen is just as beautiful as Starved Rock and usually much less busy.

GETTING THERE

CHANNAHON: From I-55, take Exit 248 onto IL 6 west into Channahon. Go 2.5 miles to Canal Street. Turn left, go 0.5 miles to Story Street and turn right into the park. If the Story Street parking area is full, continue on Canal Street one block to the Jessup Street parking area.

GEBHARD WOODS: From I-80, take Exit 112 south to Morris. Go 2 miles south on IL 47. Turn right (west) on Jefferson Street (which will turn into Fremont Street). Go 0.9 miles to Ottawa Street, turn left, and then 0.1 mile to park entrance on the left.

GPS COORDINATES

Channahon:
UTM Zone 16T
Easting 0397404
Northing 4586527
Latitude N 41° 25' 25.5212"
Longitude W 88° 13' 40.0594"

Gebhard Woods:
UTM Zone 16T
Easting 0379639
Northing 4579375
Latitude N 41° 21' 24.8077"
Longitude W 88° 26' 20.0649"

8
DELABAR
STATE PARK

DELABAR STATE PARK IS SMALL—only 89 acres— but it's perched on the banks of the largest of all the rivers that have influenced the history and geography of Illinois, the Mississippi. While this little park caters primarily to RVers, it offers a few ideal tent sites, and it's a great base from which to explore this portion of Great River Road.

After you enter Delabar, turn right, and you'll first come to the log cabin registration booth at the entrance to the Class B campground. On busy weekends the campground host may be there, or at the adjacent trailer, to register you. Otherwise, the sign will instruct you to set up your campsite, and park staff will come by later.

The entrance to the one-way campground loop is on the right, past the booth. There are 53 electric campsites, with vault toilets and water spigots throughout the campground. Most sites are spacious, though with little privacy, and usually attract RVs. For tent campers, there are two better options elsewhere in the park.

Continue north of the main campground, past the park office to the small loop on the left. Here you'll find four unnumbered nonelectric sites, two within the loop and two outside, with vault toilets and water across the road. You can park on the grass at your site. These sites don't have much shade or privacy from one another, but they are well away from the main campground.

The best spots for tent campers are the four unnumbered walk-in campsites south of the main campground. After you enter the park, turn left and drive to the parking lot at the end of the road. Vault toilets and a water spigot are to the left, and next to these is the first campsite—fairly open and just a few steps from your vehicle. Go over the hummock at the end of the lot to reveal two more sites in a spacious and well-shaded area—and best of all, hidden from view. Since they're next to each other, take one of these if you have a friend to occupy

> *Sit by the river's edge and watch the mighty Mississippi flow by.*

RATINGS

Beauty: ✯ ✯ ✯ ✯
Privacy: ✯ ✯ ✯ ✯
Spaciousness: ✯ ✯ ✯
Quiet: ✯ ✯ ✯ ✯
Security: ✯ ✯ ✯ ✯
Cleanliness: ✯ ✯ ✯ ✯ ✯

KEY INFORMATION

ADDRESS: c/o Big River State Forest, RR #1, Box 118, Keithsburg, IL

OPERATED BY: IDNR

CONTACT: (309) 374-2496, www.dnr.state.il.us/lands/Landmgt/parks/r1/delabar.htm

OPEN: Year-round

SITES: Class D: 4 walk-in tent sites; Class C: 4 sites; Class B/E: 53 sites

EACH SITE: Electric (Class B/E only); picnic table, fire ring with grill

ASSIGNMENT: Reservations accepted in person or by mail; otherwise first come, first served

REGISTRATION: Register with campground host or set up and park staff will come by

FACILITIES: Water spigots, vault toilets

PARKING: At site (Class B/E and C); at lot (Class D)

FEE: Class B: $18 per night; Class C: $8 per night; Class D: $6 per night; $5 reservation fee

ELEVATION: 566 feet

RESTRICTIONS: *Pets:* On leash only *Fires:* In fire rings only *Alcohol:* Permitted *Vehicles:* 2 per site *Other:* 14-day limit; 2 tents or 1 RV per site; 4 adults or 1 family per site

the other. The fourth site is even more concealed. Go past the single pine tree, turn right, and you'll see a picnic table back in the woods where the campsite is located. This site is smaller but more secluded, with plenty of trees and small ridges around it. Walk past the site and peer through the woods—yes, that's the mighty Mississippi you're looking down on, barely 500 feet away.

Except for holidays, Delabar is usually less than half full, but with so few walk-in sites, it's wise to reserve if you want one on a weekend. Download the general IDNR campsite reservation form from **www.dnr.state.il.us/lands/Landmgt/Programs/Camping/camprsvp.htm** and mail it in with the fee to arrive at least seven days in advance.

You can hike the woods around Delabar via two trails that begin at the main campground, covering about 2 miles. Be sure to walk down to the docks on the river's edge where you can fish or simply watch the Mississippi flow by.

Delabar is small, but nearby Big River State Forest offers 2,900 acres of largely pine woods to explore. From the entrance to Delabar, turn left and head 6.1 miles north on the Keithsburg blacktop (CR 3) to the Big River office on the right. Stop here to pick up trail maps; if the office is closed, look in the log cabin that serves as a hunter check-in station. There are hiking and equestrian trails, as well as 10 miles of designated auto routes and 30 miles of snowmobile trails. The aptly named Big Pines Trail is a beautiful 1.4-mile hiking loop; trailhead parking is about 1.2 miles south of the office on the left.

One of Illinois' few remaining fire towers is also here. If the office is open, check in to borrow the key, and climb the 60 feet to the top to look out over the Mississippi River Valley.

Big River's own Shady Pines Campground is located 0.5 miles north of the office, on the left. If the good spots at Delabar are taken, Shady Pines is a very pretty alternative, with 29 nonelectric sites situated, as you'd expect, beneath the cool cover of tall pines. Adjacent Riverview Campground was closed in 2008 due to flood damage, but if it's reopened you can camp there right along the Mississippi. Shady Pines also has a small

MAP

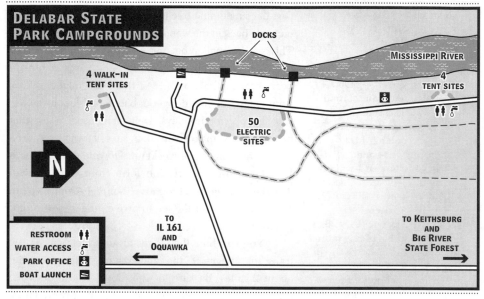

DELABAR STATE PARK CAMPGROUNDS

DOCKS

MISSISSIPPI RIVER

4 WALK-IN TENT SITES

4 TENT SITES

50 ELECTRIC SITES

N

TO IL 161 AND OQUAWKA

TO KEITHSBURG AND BIG RIVER STATE FOREST

RESTROOM	👫
WATER ACCESS	🚰
PARK OFFICE	🛈
BOAT LAUNCH	⚓

shower house, which campers from Delabar can use—have your campground permit visible on your car's dashboard.

If you're a fan of the quirky, stop by the grave of Norma Jean the elephant in nearby Oquawka. Star of a visiting circus, on July 17, 1972, Norma Jean was chained to an oak in the town square when a sudden thunderstorm came through and lightning felled both tree and elephant. Weighing in at 6,500 pounds, it was easier to bury her where she fell, and a 12-foot stone memorial marks the spot. Drive south from Delabar to the junction with IL 164, turn left, proceed 1.1 miles to Fifth Street, then turn right and go 0.4 miles.

GPS COORDINATES

UTM Zone 15T
Easting 0673288
Northing 4536125
Latitude N 40° 57' 28.4290"
Longitude W 90° 56' 27.2978"

GETTING THERE

From Monmouth, head 14.25 miles west on IL 164 to Oquawka. Turn right onto CR 3 at the Delabar sign. Proceed 1.8 miles north to another Delabar sign. Turn left and continue 0.4 miles to the park entrance.

From Milan, go 17 miles south on US 67 to IL 17 at Viola. Turn right. Proceed 19 miles to the Keithsburg sign at 76th Street. Turn left and continue 6 miles to the 4-way stop in Keithsburg. Turn left, go 0.3 miles to the next stop sign at 10th Street, turn right, and drive 10 miles to the Delabar sign. Turn right and go 0.4 miles to the park entrance.

9
WOODFORD COUNTY STATE FISH & WILDLIFE AREA

> *You can watch blue herons catch their dinner, fish for your own, or just relax at this small primitive campground near the Illinois River.*

WOODFORD COUNTY STATE FISH & WILDLIFE Area covers 2,900 acres, more than 80 percent of which is water—not surprising, since the Illinois River valley here north of Peoria is broad and low-lying, and the river spreads out to create large, shallow backwater lakes. The balance of the acreage is bottomland forest and seasonal wetlands, creating a combination that's a welcome haven for waterfowl. Equally inviting to tent campers is the small primitive campground near the river, where you can watch blue herons catch their dinner, fish for your own, or just relax.

The camping area consists of a single loop of 25 grassy sites, each with a ground grill and a table. The sites around the outside of the loop on the east are adjacent to a large field that offers plenty of space for spreading out or throwing a football. There isn't a lot of shade, but sites 1 and 2 have some pines, and 6 and 8, at the back of the loop, are the best-shaded and nicest sites. The west side of the loop is bordered by a man-made fishing channel that connects to the river. You'll find vault toilets and a water spigot at the end of the loop. The only RV you'll probably see is the one in the middle of the loop, belonging to the campground host. Register with the host; if no one is there, park staff will come by.

There's nothing fancy or particularly scenic about the campground itself. What is attractive is the quiet. Outside of waterfowl-hunting season (when the campground is closed), not many people make the 1-mile drive off IL 26 to this secluded spot along the river. In April and May, a very busy weekend might see half the sites occupied; during the summer and early fall, chances are good it will just be you and the campground host. Note that the campground is only open from April 1 to October 1.

RATINGS

Beauty: ✩ ✩ ✩
Privacy: ✩ ✩ ✩
Spaciousness: ✩ ✩ ✩
Quiet: ✩ ✩ ✩ ✩ ✩
Security: ✩ ✩ ✩ ✩
Cleanliness: ✩ ✩ ✩ ✩

You can't see the Illinois River from your campsite, but you can walk or drive about 0.25 miles to it, and the view is impressive. The river spreads out across the lowlands to form shallow Goose Lake, and the opposite shore is about 2 miles away at this point. There's a boat ramp and fish-cleaning station here. There are also three hiking trails starting at the end of the campground and extending about 1 mile north. The hiking is easy, with trails following along the tops of the levees created to manage seasonal flooding of the wetlands. The westernmost, Goose Lake Trail, offers the best views of the river. You can hike that out, and pick up Wood Duck Trail for the return trip, making a 2-mile loop.

Bird-watchers like this area along the Illinois River because of the abundance of waterfowl, raptors, and many other species. You'll certainly see wood ducks, Canada geese, blue herons, egrets, swans, red-tailed hawks, owls, and, if you're fortunate, bald eagles. They're more common in the winter, but in 2007 and 2008 a nesting pair of bald eagles was located about 1.5 miles south of nearby Marshall State Fish & Wildlife Area, between the highway and the river. Park staff built a short trail and viewing blind so visitors could watch without disturbing them. There's no guarantee the eagles will return, but check with the ranger at Marshall, which oversees Woodford.

Marshall is 5.8 miles north of Woodford on IL 26, also right on the Illinois River. There's a small campground there and, unlike Woodford's, it's open year-round. This spot tends to attract more campers, probably because it has 22 electric sites and is visible from the highway. Some of the electric sites on the west side (notably sites 5 through 11) are well shaded and offer a beautiful view of the river. There are also six sandy non-electric sites bunched together, and toilets and a water spigot are. The biggest drawback to camping at Marshall is the highway noise—the campsites are barely 150 feet from IL 26. A fence separates the electric sites from the highway, but nothing shields the non-electric ones.

Just across IL 26, to the east, the land quickly rises some 200 feet in impressive wooded bluffs. Marshall includes 3.5 miles of fairly rugged trails that traverse this upland oak-hickory forest, winding along the bluffs

KEY INFORMATION

ADDRESS:	524 Conservation Lane, Lowpoint, IL 61545
OPERATED BY:	IDNR
CONTACT:	c/o Marshall SFWA (309) 246-8351, www.dnr.state.il.us/lands/landmgt/parks/r1/woodford.htm
OPEN:	Apr. 1–Oct. 1
SITES:	25 Class C sites
EACH SITE:	Picnic table, ground grill
ASSIGNMENT:	First come, first served
REGISTRATION:	Register with campground host or set up and park staff will come by
FACILITIES:	Water spigots, vault toilets
PARKING:	At campsite
FEE:	$8 per night
ELEVATION:	444 feet
RESTRICTIONS:	*Pets:* On leash only *Fires:* In fire rings only *Alcohol:* Permitted *Vehicles:* 2 per site *Other:* 14-day limit; 4 adults or 1 family per site

MAP

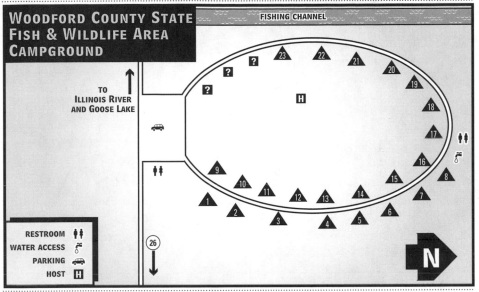

WOODFORD COUNTY STATE FISH & WILDLIFE AREA CAMPGROUND

FISHING CHANNEL

TO ILLINOIS RIVER AND GOOSE LAKE

RESTROOM
WATER ACCESS
PARKING
HOST

GETTING THERE

From I-74 at East Peoria, take Exit 95 to IL 116 and head north 5 miles to IL 26. Take the left fork onto IL 26, and go 12.6 miles to Conservation Lane. Turn left, and drive 0.9 miles to the campground entrance.

From I-39, take Exit 35 to IL 17, then head west 18.3 miles to IL 26 in Lacon. Turn left, go 10.5 miles south to Conservation Lane, make a right, and drive 0.9 miles to the campground entrance.

and up and down the ravines. I don't think many people take advantage of these beautiful trails. I suggest hiking the loop clockwise—start with the moderate 0.5-mile walk down to the bluffs on Walnut Trail, then take your time enjoying the views along the 0.75-mile Bluff Trail, and finish getting a workout on the 2-mile Ravine Run Trail, with its staircases and bridges. To get to the trailhead, go 1 mile north of the Marshall entrance, then turn right onto Richland Road. Continue 0.5 miles to Blue Heron Road and turn right. Go 0.6 miles to the trailhead parking on the right. Pick up a trail map at the Marshall office, north of the campground, on the east side of the highway.

GPS COORDINATES

UTM Zone 16T
Easting 0293388
Northing 4528224
Latitude N 40° 52' 44.5397"
Longitude W 89° 27' 7.6086"

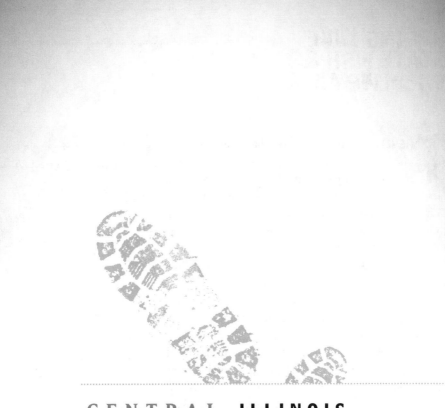

CENTRAL ILLINOIS

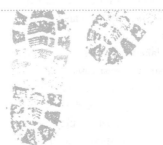

10
SPRING LAKE STATE FISH & WILDLIFE AREA

THE ILLINOIS RIVER VALLEY has been attracting visitors for over 10,000 years, when the first Native Americans settled there to take advantage of the abundant wildlife, water, and fertile soil. Today a number of parks and wildlife refuges continue to draw hunters, anglers, birders, and campers to the area. One of the prettiest places to camp is beneath the oak or pine trees at Spring Lake State Fish & Wildlife Area. The park offers two quite different camping areas, separated from each other by several miles, and ample opportunities for wildlife viewing and fishing.

The narrow, shallow lake that makes up two-thirds of Spring Lake's 2,032 acres is an abandoned channel of the Illinois River and runs parallel to the river for about 8 miles on its eastern side. These are the river's bottomlands, but the lake is bordered on the east by a large sandstone bluff, and the park's campgrounds, office, and hiking trails are on that side, about 80 feet above the lake level. The lake is divided into northern and southern sections by an east–west causeway.

The walk-in camping area is at the southern end of the lake, near the office. Register and park there, then cross the road to one of the six sites—three close to the road, and three up on the grass-covered hill. The sites are spread out, though they don't have much shade or brush between them. I suggest walking the extra distance for the sites farthest out, as the others are within sight of the park maintenance building—kind of like camping near a garage. Each site has a picnic table and a fire ring; there are vault toilets nearby, and there's a water spigot by the road. This area also doubles as the group campground, used by youth groups about ten weekends a year. Though not required to do so, most groups notify the office in advance, so you can ask if any are scheduled before deciding to camp there.

> *Camp beneath towering pines, with a bed of soft pine needles under your tent.*

RATINGS

Beauty: ☆ ☆ ☆
Privacy: ☆ ☆ ☆
Spaciousness: ☆ ☆ ☆
Quiet: ☆ ☆ ☆ ☆
Security: ☆ ☆ ☆ ☆
Cleanliness: ☆ ☆ ☆ ☆ ☆

KEY INFORMATION

As a tent camper, my first inclination is to go for the walk-in sites—I assume they'll be more secluded, more attractive, and less used. At Spring Lake, however, I prefer the vehicular access sites at the northern end of the lake. They're much prettier, well shaded, and usually not busy. From the office, head 3.25 miles north to the causeway, cross the lake, and continue 1.75 miles on Spring Lake Road to the northern campground entrance, on the left. One-quarter mile in you'll come to an intersection and have to make a choice: Oak Campground on the right, or Pine Campground on the left? Both are aptly named. The 38 sites along the Oak loop sit beneath spreading oaks, with a few pines thrown in and some trees and brush separating the sites from one another. Head toward the back of the loop, where the sites are roomier—I like 18 and 20.

Pine is the smaller of the two loops, with 22 sites, and is definitely my favorite place to camp at Spring Lake. It's a rare treat to camp beneath towering pines in Illinois—I love the scent and the bed of soft pine needles under the tent. Some sites on the northern outside of the loop are a bit hilly, but the rest are excellent. Site 51, at the far end, probably offers the most space and distance from neighboring sites. Site 60, on the left near the entrance, is also larger, and 57 and 58, while smaller, are tucked away from view.

All sites have a table and a fire ring, and there are water spigots and vault toilets nearby. Just pitch your tent, and park staff will come by to register you later. You'll never have trouble finding a spot here—the campground never completely fills up, even on holiday weekends. On most fair-weather non-holiday weekends, about one-third of the 60 sites will be occupied, whether by tents or by smaller RVs.

Fishing is a prime attraction at Spring Lake, particularly in the spring, before the growth of aquatic vegetation makes it more challenging. The north lake is better suited to boat fishing, and largemouth bass and muskie are among the targets. The south lake has plenty of well-mown spots for bank fishing, and these can be accessed from the six parking areas along the 2-mile stretch of road from the causeway south. Besides the typical bass, bluegill, crappie, and channel catfish, south

MAP

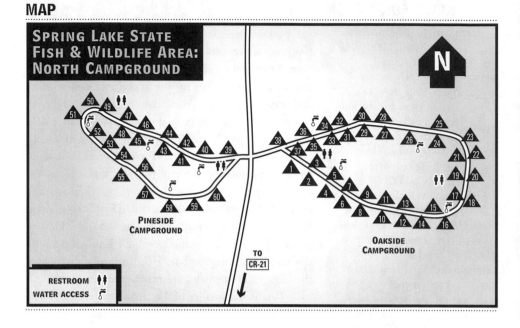

lake's cool spring-fed waters support a healthy population of northern pike. There's a nice picnic area at the southern end of the lake and a fish-cleaning station at the boat ramp along the causeway.

For food, boat rental, bait, or just simple advice on what's biting where, head to Larry's Restaurant and Bar, on the southern lake, 2 miles south of the causeway. The menu offers sandwiches and snacks until 3 p.m., then serves dinner, offering specials on the weekends. Larry's is open Wednesday through Sunday, except in winter, from 8 a.m. to 10 p.m. (8 p.m. on Sundays). Boats (without motors) are available from May 1 to mid-October. Phone (309) 968-9500 for more information.

GETTING THERE

From Pekin, take IL 29 south about 1 mile to Manito Road. Turn right (west) and go 10.3 miles to Spring Lake Road. Turn right again and travel 3.1 miles west to the north campground entrance, on the right. To get to the office, continue west on Spring Lake Road 1.75 miles across the lake, turn left, and go 3.25 miles south.

GPS COORDINATES

North Campground Entrance:
UTM Zone 16T
Easting 0259004
Northing 4483251
Latitude N 40° 27' 54.0100"
Longitude W 89° 50' 32.9694"

11
SAND RIDGE
STATE FOREST

> *Explore miles of forest trails in Illinois' desert, complete with prickly pear cactus.*

FOR A STATE PRESUMED TO BE ALL CORNFIELD, Illinois boasts an amazing diversity of habitat: wetlands and forests, bluffs and meadows, canyons, and a wealth of lakes and rivers. One expanse of wilderness southwest of Peoria is even reminiscent of the desert. Sand Ridge State Forest sits atop 7,500 acres of sandy soil, about half oak–hickory forest, one-third pine, and much of the rest sand prairie. At the close of the last ice age, the receding floodwaters left a vast amount of sand through this portion of the Illinois River valley. The winds sculpted the 100-foot dunes that became the wooded ridges the area is named for. This unique environment supports plant and animal species more typical of the Southwest than the Midwest, including prickly pear cactus.

Sand Ridge is also a great place to hike and camp if you want quiet and miles of forest trails to explore. As you enter on CR 2300 North, you'll find Pine Campground at the crossroads with Cactus Drive, situated within the shade of a beautiful grove of tall pines. Water spigots and vault toilets are conveniently located, and each site has a table and a ground grill. Over the holidays it may be close to full, but most other weekends you won't have more than a handful of neighbors.

The 23 sites are laid out in three small loops, labeled A, B, and C, from east to west. A few sites are a bit small or too close to adjacent sites, but most are otherwise good choices. I prefer the sites on the outside and back of each loop because they tend to be larger and better shaded and those in loop C because it's farther from the campground entrance. Site C5 is tucked away in its own bit of woods; B6 is my favorite—it's off the road and is the most spacious.

Sand Ridge also has 12 secluded hike-in campsites scattered throughout the forest; the closest is about 0.25 miles from the nearest parking. Each has a fire

RATINGS

Beauty: ✿ ✿ ✿ ✿
Privacy: ✿ ✿ ✿ ✿ ✿
Spaciousness: ✿ ✿ ✿
Quiet: ✿ ✿ ✿ ✿ ✿
Security: ✿ ✿ ✿ ✿
Cleanliness: ✿ ✿ ✿ ✿ ✿

ring but no water or other facilities. Most are in wooded settings, out of sight of the trail, and have enough room for several tents. Before camping, you must register at the park office, open 8 a.m. to 4 p.m. daily. If you arrive after office hours, camp at Pine Campground the first night and arrange for hike-in camping the next day. You can park at the lot closest to your site, or along the road, as long as you don't block a fire lane. Pick up a trail map from the Web site or forest staff, and check with them on the status of individual sites and the best place to park for closest access.

One attractive wooded hike-in site is BC 4, located on a small hill and off the trail. To get there, go 0.4 miles south from the crossroads of CR 2300 and Cactus Drive. Park off the road, and pick up the red trail on the west side of the road. After about 700 feet you come to the junction with the orange trail; turn right, and continue another 2,000 feet to the campsite, on the left, a total hike of about 0.5 miles.

Whether you want a little hiking or a lot, you'll find something suitable at Sand Ridge. The woods and interspersed meadows are beautiful and quiet. In the late spring or early summer, you may see the abundant prickly pear cactus in bloom, with their waxy yellow flowers. The fall offers the changing leaves, in all their colorful radiance. With about 44 miles of trail available, you can hike all day and rarely meet another person. The trail system is composed of seven interconnecting loops, each blazed in a different color. The shortest loop is 1.25 miles long, and the longest is about 17 miles, with all sorts of possible routes between them. If that's not enough, there are also more than 120 miles of unmarked fire lanes that are not on the trail map—bring a compass or GPS if you want to hike these. Otherwise, stick to the trails, and remember that they'll cross the wider fire lanes at various points. Note that most of the trail system may also be shared by equestrians—the 2-mile green loop and the backcountry campsites are closed to horses.

The biggest challenge in hiking at Sand Ridge is the sand. The terrain is fairly level, but the sandy soil makes walking much more strenuous. Plan accordingly, and bring plenty of water. Hiking along the trail edge

KEY INFORMATION

ADDRESS:	25799 East CR 2300 North, P.O. Box 111, Forest City, IL 61532
OPERATED BY:	IDNR
CONTACT:	(309) 597-2212, www.dnr.state.il .us/lands/land mgt/parks/r4/ sand.htm
OPEN:	Year-round (except firearm deer season, late Nov.–early Dec.)
SITES:	Class C: 23 sites; Class D: 12 hike-in sites; Class C equestrian: 20 sites
EACH SITE:	Table, ground grill
ASSIGNMENT:	First come, first served
REGISTRATION:	Register at the office
FACILITIES:	Water spigot, vault toilets at Class C campsites only
PARKING:	At campsite; nearest parking lot or roadside (hike-in sites)
FEE:	Class C: $8 per night; Class D: $6 per night
ELEVATION:	499 feet
RESTRICTIONS:	*Pets:* On leash only *Fires:* In fire rings only *Alcohol:* Not permitted *Vehicles:* 2 per site

MAP

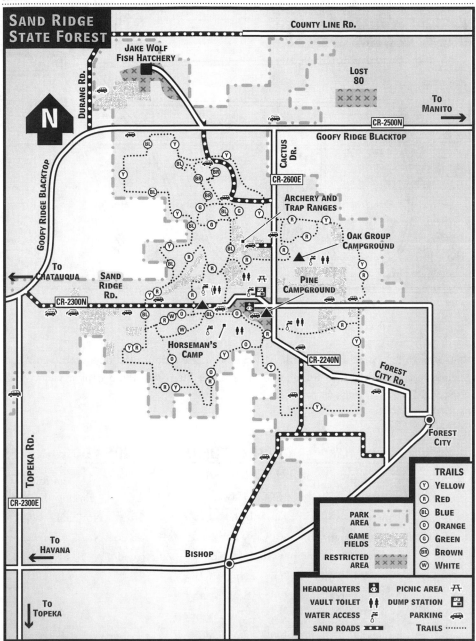

SAND RIDGE STATE FOREST

JAKE WOLF FISH HATCHERY

COUNTY LINE RD.

DURANG RD.

LOST 80

TO MANITO

N

CR-2500N

GOOFY RIDGE BLACKTOP

GOOFY RIDGE BLACKTOP

CACTUS DR.

CR-2600E

ARCHERY AND TRAP RANGES

OAK GROUP CAMPGROUND

TO CHATAUQUA

SAND RIDGE RD.

CR-2300N

PINE CAMPGROUND

HORSEMAN'S CAMP

CR-2240N

FOREST CITY RD.

FOREST CITY

TOPEKA RD.

CR-2300E

TO HAVANA

BISHOP

TO TOPEKA

TRAILS	
Ⓨ	YELLOW
Ⓡ	RED
ⓑ	BLUE
ⓞ	ORANGE
Ⓖ	GREEN
ⓑⓡ	BROWN
Ⓦ	WHITE

PARK AREA	
GAME FIELDS	
RESTRICTED AREA	

HEADQUARTERS		PICNIC AREA	
VAULT TOILET		DUMP STATION	
WATER ACCESS		PARKING	
SAND ROADS		TRAILS	

provides firmer footing in places. Watch for indentations in the sand made by horses' hooves, which can be ankle-twisters.

There's no fishing at Sand Ridge—water doesn't stay on the surface long enough to even make a mud puddle—but you can tour the state's largest fish hatchery. The Jake Wolff Memorial Fish Hatchery operates year-round and is open Monday through Friday from

MAP

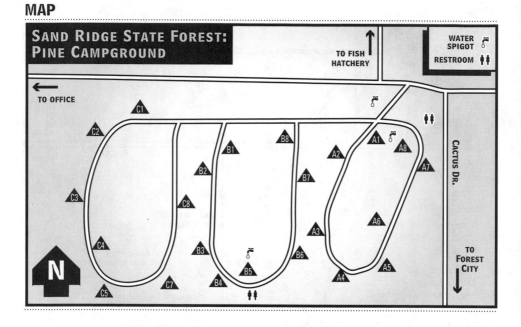

SAND RIDGE STATE FOREST: PINE CAMPGROUND

TO FISH HATCHERY

WATER SPIGOT

RESTROOM

TO OFFICE

CACTUS DR.

TO FOREST CITY

N

C1 C2 C3 C4 C5 C7 C8 B1 B2 B3 B4 B5 B6 B7 B8 A1 A2 A3 A4 A5 A6 A7 A8

8:30 a.m. to 3:30 p.m. The upper level visitor center overlooks the operation below and features various exhibits on fishing and the pioneer life of the Illinois River valley. Call (309) 968-7531 to arrange a visit.

GETTING THERE

From east or west, take US 136 to CR 2800 East (12 miles east of Havana or 20 miles west of I-155). Turn north and go 6 miles straight, through Forest City. The road turns west and becomes CR 2300 North. Continue 2 miles to Pine Campground. From the Peoria area, follow IL 29 south from Pekin to Manito Road. Turn right (west) and go 13.5 miles south into Manito. Turn right again onto CR 2500 North (Goofy Ridge Road). Drive 4.1 miles to Cactus Drive, then turn left (south) and go 2 miles to Pine Campground.

GPS COORDINATES

UTM Zone 16T
Easting 0256698
Northing 4475071
Latitude N 40° 23' 26.6251"
Longitude W 89° 51' 59.4958"

THE BEST IN TENT CAMPING ILLINOIS

> *COMLARA offers some excellent, serene, and even secluded spots for tent campers.*

COMLARA PARK IS BOTH BEAUTIFUL and busy. McLean County has developed an attractive, well-maintained, and well-staffed recreational getaway here around 700-acre Evergreen Lake. The facilities are superb and the grounds manicured. Even the shower house is among the nicest I've seen in any campground. And with Bloomington–Normal's 110,000 people just to the south, it's also very popular with locals, who come to enjoy camping, boating, fishing, swimming, and trail biking. Despite this, COMLARA offers some serene and even secluded spots for tent campers in this excellent park.

Enter the park off CR 33, and stop at the visitor center on the left. If you don't have a reservation, you'll need to register here first. (After hours, you can use the self-registration post at the main campground entrance.) You can also pick up a park map and brochures on hiking, camping, or fishing, and purchase firewood and ice if you need them.

Turn right at the office, and enter the campground. Yes, it's big (130 sites), and probably full of RVs, but keep heading straight back. Continue past the shower house, curving left and to the back of the campground. Just past site 107 you'll reach the first of two parking areas for the 11 walk-in tent sites. The second is about 1,000 feet down the road, past site 114. The grass-covered sites are a short walk from parking, and each has a picnic table, fire ring, and scenic views of Evergreen Lake.

Site 126, the first you encounter, is beautiful and right on the lake. Surrounded by trees, it feels at least a little private, even if the rest of the campground is crowded. Sites 122, 123, and 125 are good; 124 is too small, and 118, 119, 120, and 121 are too open and close to each other. Sites 119B and 120B are my other first choices—close to the water, with trees and brush

RATINGS

Beauty: ✪ ✪ ✪ ✪
Privacy: ✪ ✪
Spaciousness: ✪ ✪ ✪
Quiet: ✪ ✪ ✪ ✪
Security: ✪ ✪ ✪ ✪
Cleanliness: ✪ ✪ ✪ ✪ ✪

separating them from their neighbors. Since you can reserve any site at COMLARA, I recommend spending the extra $6 to hold one of these. Reservations can be made in person starting the first Saturday in April, and by mail or phone the Monday following.

If the main campground is too busy for you, and you don't mind walking a bit, you will love the White Oak primitive area on the other side of the lake. Go first to the visitor center to register, then head out of the park, turn left on CR 33, and turn left again on CR 8 at the stop sign. Continue 3.75 miles around the lake to the next stop sign. Turn left and go 0.75 miles. Head past the wooden White Oak group camping signboard on the right, then watch for a grassy area by a gate on the right. Though there's no sign, this is the walk-in parking. Walk past the gate and the vault toilets and watch carefully for the trail signs. These eight sites are right on the edge of the lake, each tucked away in its own little wooded enclave, completely separate from the others. Site 5 is very private, site 3 has its own dock, and site 10 is the largest. Site 8 is a bit small and sloped; the only drawback to site 4 is that you have to walk through it to get to site 3. You'll have to walk about 0.3 miles to get from your vehicle to the farthest sites, 3 and 10, but the peace, privacy, and beauty of these spots make it well worth the effort. If you have your own boat, you can actually pull right up to all but sites 5, 6, and 7 from the lake. (The Web site says there are ten walk-in sites; at press time, however, accessible sites A1 and A2 had not yet been developed.)

Water is available back at the main campground entrance, and you can use the shower house there. The White Oak sites are open from the first Saturday in April through October 15. Surprisingly, they also book up well in advance on the weekends, so it's wise to make reservations. Even with a reservation, be sure you stop at the visitor center when you arrive—or the next morning at the latest—to get a vehicle tag.

COMLARA boasts plenty of recreational opportunities, including more than 10 miles of trails for mountain biking and hiking, along with fishing, boating, and swimming. To reach the beach and main boat-launch area, turn left at the park entrance and pass the

KEY INFORMATION

ADDRESS: RR 1, COMLARA Park Rd., Hudson, IL 61748

OPERATED BY: McLean County Dept. of Parks & Recreation

CONTACT: (309) 726-2022 (ext. 221), www.mclean countyil.gov/parks /camping.htm

OPEN: Year-round (main campground); Apr. 1–Oct. 15 (White Oak)

SITES: 93 electric; 25 non-electric; 11 walk-in (main camp-ground); 8 walk-in (White Oak)

EACH SITE: Electric (93 sites); picnic table, fire ring

ASSIGNMENT: Reservations available

REGISTRATION: At visitor center; at self-registration post after hours

FACILITIES: Water spigots, vault toilets, shower house

PARKING: At site, or in lot

FEE: $14 per night (non-electric), $20 per night (50 amp), $17 per night (30 amp); $6 reservation fee

ELEVATION: 746 feet

RESTRICTIONS: *Pets:* On leash only
Fires: In fire rings only
Alcohol: Not permitted
Vehicles: 2 per site
Other: 14-day limit; 1 RV or 2 tents per site; no more than 8 people per site; collecting of firewood prohibited

MAP

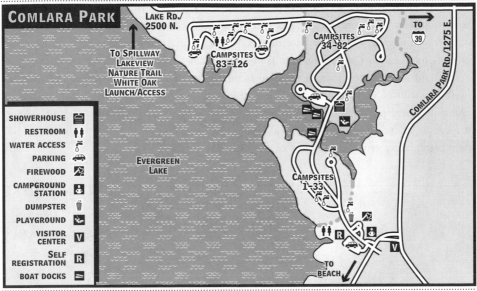

COMLARA PARK

Lake Rd./ 2500 N.

To Spillway Lakeview Nature Trail White Oak Launch/Access

CAMPSITES 83–126

CAMPSITES 34–82

TO 39

COMLARA PARK RD./1275 E.

EVERGREEN LAKE

CAMPSITES 1–33

SHOWERHOUSE	
RESTROOM	
WATER ACCESS	
PARKING	
FIREWOOD	
CAMPGROUND STATION	
DUMPSTER	
PLAYGROUND	
VISITOR CENTER	V
SELF REGISTRATION	R
BOAT DOCKS	

R

V

TO BEACH

MAP

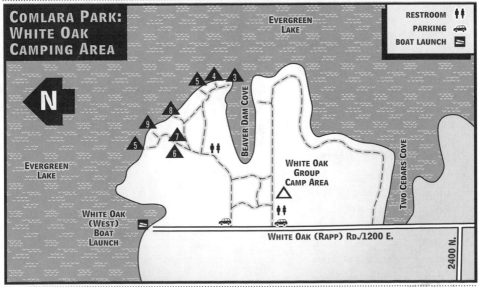

COMLARA PARK: WHITE OAK CAMPING AREA

RESTROOM	
PARKING	
BOAT LAUNCH	

EVERGREEN LAKE

N

5 4 3

8

9

5

7

6

BEAVER DAM COVE

WHITE OAK GROUP CAMP AREA

TWO CEDARS COVE

EVERGREEN LAKE

WHITE OAK (WEST) BOAT LAUNCH

WHITE OAK (RAPP) RD./1200 E.

2400 N.

visitor center. The beachfront is actually on a separate 2.5-acre lake ringed with 4 acres of sandy beach. It features deep and shallow areas, a diving platform, a giant water umbrella, float-tube rental, showers, lockers, a playground, and a concession area. The beach is open daily from mid-May to the first Saturday in August, from noon to 5:30 p.m., and on weekends through Labor Day. A lifeguard is always on duty.

Right next to the beach is the boat launch. You can rent paddleboats, canoes, and rowboats with or without a motor. Check the Web site for rates on the beach and boat rental. If you're planning a weekend trip to COMLARA, you should also check the Web site events calendar. COMLARA occasionally hosts special events during the summer that may bring larger crowds, and parts of the lake may be closed.

GETTING THERE

From Bloomington, take I-39 north 8 miles to Exit 8 for CR 8. Go left (west) 1.5 miles on CR 8, then turn left on COMLARA Road (CR 33). Go 0.5 miles to the park entrance, on the left.

GPS COORDINATES

UTM Zone 16T
Easting 0328375
Northing 4501106
Latitude N 40° 38' 34.7352"
Longitude W 89° 1' 46.9519"

> *The prime attraction of the ten Tall Timber campsites is their seclusion from one another.*

AT MORAINE VIEW STATE RECREATION AREA, you can view something very old and something very new. Approaching the park from the south, you'll see a long high rampart running east to west. The park sits atop this end moraine, a ridge of earth and rock that was left behind by the glaciers as they retreated north at the end of the last Ice Age, some 20,000 years ago.

Once you get atop the moraine, scan the horizon to the north and east, and you'll be able to see some of the 240 white wind turbine generators of the Twin Groves Wind Farm, completed in 2007.

Besides the geology and technology, Moraine View offers some good camping options, as well as fishing, hiking, swimming, and boating. While the 137-site Gander Bay RV campground fills up virtually every weekend during camping season, the walk-in campgrounds are a better choice for tent campers and not as busy.

If you want to park close to your campsite and don't mind the possibility of having neighbors, choose among the 22 walk-in sites at the Catfish Bay Tent area. Sites 21 and 22 are closest to parking (less than 100 feet away), and those farthest (sites 11 and 12) require a hike of only about 350 feet.

Catfish Bay is on a small hill, is moderately shaded, and overlooks the lake. The sites are somewhat open to one another, and the ground slopes toward the water in places. Each site has a table and ground grill; you'll find water and the vault toilets in the parking lot. Sites 1 and 2 are wheelchair accessible and are only open to other campers if unoccupied after 8 p.m., and then only for one night. If you want space and no slope, site 3 is great. If you prefer a bit more distance and foliage between you and the neighbors, sites 16 and 18 are

RATINGS

Beauty: ☆ ☆ ☆ ☆
Privacy: ☆ ☆ ☆ ☆ ☆
Spaciousness: ☆ ☆ ☆
Quiet: ☆ ☆ ☆ ☆
Security: ☆ ☆ ☆ ☆
Cleanliness: ☆ ☆ ☆ ☆

good. I like camping by the water's edge, so sites 9 and 11 are my first choices.

Unfortunately, even these walk-in sites will be full on a holiday weekend; they can even fill up on regular weekends during good weather. They're not reservable, so plan to arrive early.

If you prefer more solitude and don't mind hiking a bit, check out the Tall Timber backpacking area. The prime attraction of these ten sites, shaded by mature hardwoods, is their seclusion from one another. These sites are the last to go on a busy weekend, and even if they're all occupied, you won't see your neighbors. Laid out in a 1.5-mile loop in the woods, each site has a table and a fire ring. The longest hike in this area is to site 6 (about 0.5 miles), but the other sites are much closer. Start at the parking lot, where the self-registration signboard will show you which sites are open. Go right (counterclockwise) around the loop, and you'll reach site 1 in about 800 feet. And if you have more gear than you want to lug even that distance, you can pull off to the side of the road closest to site 1 (you'll see the picnic table through the woods), carry everything to the site, and then go park at the trailhead. The only disadvantage to site 1 is its proximity to the road—it's a little harder to imagine yourself alone in the wilderness with the sound of the occasional car going by.

All of the Tall Timber sites offer plenty of space and shade, but my favorite is site 10, both because it's not a long walk (less than 1,000 feet) and because it's a little different from the others. From the parking area, hike straight ahead (south) about 250 feet until you see the first side trail to the left. This junction isn't well marked, so you'll have to watch for it. Turn left and head east and southeast about 700 feet. Site 10 is perched above the banks of Salt Creek and is close enough to the end of the lake that you can just hear the water tumbling over the dam. If this is music to your ears, this spot's perfect for you.

Moraine View also features a concession, near the boat dock, which offers boat rentals and sells tackle, bait, snacks, and some supplies. The restaurant serves breakfast and lunch, and you can eat on the patio

KEY INFORMATION

ADDRESS:	27374 Moraine View Park Road, LeRoy, IL 61752
OPERATED BY:	IDNR
CONTACT:	(309) 724-8032, www.dnr.state.il.us/lands/landmgt/parks/r3/moraine.htm
OPEN:	Year-round
SITES:	Class D: 22 walk-in and 10 backpacking sites; Class A: 137 RV sites and 30 equestrian sites
EACH SITE:	Electric in Class A only; picnic table, grill, fire block
ASSIGNMENT:	First come, first served; 61 Class A sites reservable by mail
REGISTRATION:	With campground host (Class A); self-registration (Class D)
FACILITIES:	Water spigots, vault toilets; shower house (Class A only, closed Nov. 1–mid-Apr.)
PARKING:	At campsite (Class A); at trailhead (Class D)
FEE:	Class D: $6 per night; Class A: $20 per night, $30 per night on holidays; $5 reservation fee
ELEVATION:	851 feet
RESTRICTIONS:	*Pets:* On leash only *Fires:* In fire rings only *Alcohol:* Not permitted in campgrounds *Vehicles:* 2 per site *Other:* 14-day limit

MAP

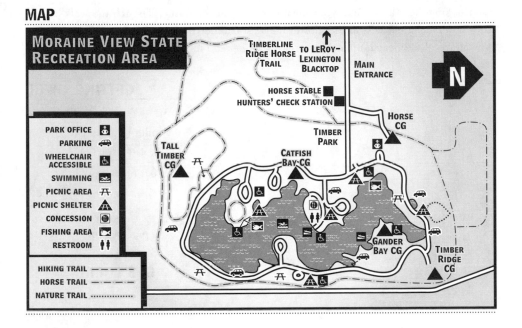

MORAINE VIEW STATE RECREATION AREA

Timberline Ridge Horse Trail

to LeRoy-Lexington Blacktop

Main Entrance

N

Horse Stable
Hunters' Check Station

Timber Park

Horse CG

Tall Timber CG

Catfish Bay CG

Gander Bay CG

Timber Ridge CG

PARK OFFICE	
PARKING	
WHEELCHAIR ACCESSIBLE	
SWIMMING	
PICNIC AREA	
PICNIC SHELTER	
CONCESSION	
FISHING AREA	
RESTROOM	

HIKING TRAIL — — —
HORSE TRAIL —·—·—
NATURE TRAIL ············

MAP

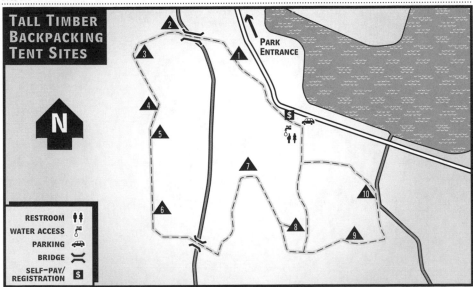

TALL TIMBER BACKPACKING TENT SITES

Park Entrance

N

RESTROOM	
WATER ACCESS	
PARKING	
BRIDGE	
SELF-PAY/ REGISTRATION	

overlooking the lake or take your meal back to your campsite. Though the walk-in tent sites don't include access to the shower house at Gander Bay, for $1 per day you can take advantage of the beach, open Memorial Day weekend to Labor Day.

GETTING THERE

From I-74 at Exit 149, head 0.5 miles north to US 150 in LeRoy. Turn left. Continue 0.6 miles to West Street (CR 21). Turn right, and go 4.1 miles north to park sign on the right.

GPS COORDINATES

UTM Zone 16T
Easting 0353482
Northing 4474867
Latitude N 40° 24' 48.2"
Longitude W 88° 43' 36.5"

14
SILOAM SPRINGS
STATE PARK

> *Let your impatient younger anglers try out the Kids Pond, where catches of 10–15 fish per half hour are common.*

RARELY HAVE I HAD TO STOP FOR DEER more frequently in Illinois than I did driving through Siloam Springs State Park. With 3,323 acres, there's plenty of room for wildlife, and white-tailed deer and wild turkey are a common sight. The four main campgrounds at Siloam Springs also provide plenty of options for campers, who can spread out and choose the setting that best suits them.

As you enter the park, take the first right and pass the group campground to reach Hickory Hill Campground. To me, these 33 sites are not as attractive as those in the Pine Grove and Oak Ridge campgrounds— but they're also not as busy. If you want fewer neighbors and don't mind driving to the showers, this is a good place. Here you'll find more singles and couples camping, and fewer families.

Most of these sites are electric, and, peculiar to Siloam Springs, tents at electric sites must be pitched on the square gravel tent pads, not on the grass. This does provide a nice, flat, raised surface, but I prefer natural earth beneath my tent. Fortunately, Hickory Hill features 11 non-electric grass tent sites on the south side of this elongated loop, set off in three sections up against the woods. You can't park at each site, but the farthest is only about 50 feet away. Circle the loop counterclockwise, and you'll come first to my favorite set of sites, 9B, 10B, and 11B. There's plenty of space, and you're as far from other campers as you can be here. Site 11B is the most popular, well shaded by two massive oak trees. It's also right by the 0.25-mile Raccoon Trail, which leads down to a floating dock on the lake, where you can fish or simply sit and watch the sun rise. Don't pitch your tent right by the trailhead, though, unless you like having other campers trudge through your campsite.

If any of these first three sites is taken, move down to the next set, 6B through 8B, or the third, 1B through

RATINGS

Beauty: ✩ ✩ ✩
Privacy: ✩ ✩ ✩
Spaciousness: ✩ ✩ ✩
Quiet: ✩ ✩ ✩ ✩
Security: ✩ ✩ ✩ ✩
Cleanliness: ✩ ✩ ✩ ✩ ✩

5B. On an average non-holiday weekend you have a good chance of getting one of these sections to yourself.

Another alternative for tent campers is the group campground, which you pass on the way to Hickory Hill. When they're not reserved or occupied by a group, individuals can pick one of the 30 or so unnumbered non-electric sites in this grassy area. These aren't as well shaded as the ones in Hickory Hill, but if you want more privacy this is a good choice. The weekend I camped at Hickory Hill, there was one lone camper in the group area. Note that Hickory Hill and the group campground are closed from November 1 to April 1.

Farther into the park, you'll find the entrance to Pine Grove and Oak Ridge campgrounds, along the same road. These are busier, with more RVs, but they're also more scenic and closer to the showers. As you drive in, Pine Grove is particularly striking, with well-laid-out sites set beneath tall, stately pines. Of the 76 sites in these two areas, 16 are designated tent-only, and 12 of these are electric, scattered among the RV sites: in the first loop they are 9, 10, 11, 14, 16, 17, and 24; in the second, 41 and 56; and in the third, 71, 80, and 81. If you want electricity, the most attractive and spacious of these are 9, 10, and 11. However, to me the nicest for tent camping are the non-electric sites 61 to 64, all by themselves down the road in Oak Ridge. Each has a table, fire ring, lantern pole, and tent pad.

Fishing is a prime draw at Siloam Springs, particularly at the start of the trout seasons, the first Saturday in April and the third Saturday in October. You can bank or boat fish, or cast a line from one of the six floating docks around the 58-acre lake. The concession sells bait, tackle, ice, firewood, and some snacks, and rents paddleboats and rowboats with trolling motors. They're usually open every day but Wednesday from April 1 to November 1, 8 a.m. to 6 p.m. (Saturdays from 7 a.m. to 7 p.m.). Phone (217) 894-6271 for more information.

If you have impatient younger anglers, let them test the waters at the Kids Pond, right by the park entrance. They can bank fish almost all the way around the pond, and catches of 10 to 15 redear and bluegill per half hour are common.

KEY INFORMATION

ADDRESS: 938 East 3003rd Lane, Clayton, IL

OPERATED BY: IDNR

CONTACT: (217) 894-6205, www.dnr.state.il.us/lands/landmgt/parks/r4/siloamsp.htm

OPEN: Year-round

SITES: Class B: 46 non-electric sites; Class A: 83 electric sites; 4 backpacking sites; 28 equestrian-only sites

EACH SITE: Picnic table, ground grill; electric at Class A only

ASSIGNMENT: First come, first served

REGISTRATION: Select site, then register with campground host or office

FACILITIES: Water spigots, vault toilets; shower house (closed mid-Dec.–Apr. 1)

PARKING: At site; in lot (walk-in sites); at park office (backpacking sites)

FEE: Class A: $20 per night, $30 per night holidays; Class B: $10 per night; backpacking: $8 per night

ELEVATION: 684 feet

RESTRICTIONS: *Pets:* On leash only *Fires:* In fire rings only *Alcohol:* Permitted *Vehicles:* 2 per site *Other:* 14-day limit; 1 RV and 1 tent, or 2 tents per site; 4 adults or 1 family per site

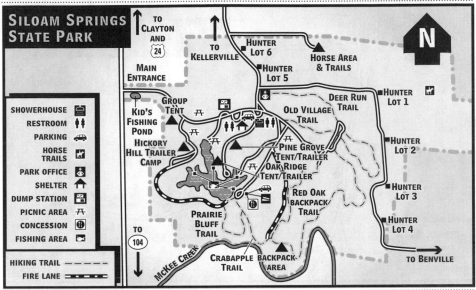

SILOAM SPRINGS STATE PARK

TO CLAYTON AND US 24

TO KELLERVILLE

Main Entrance

Hunter Lot 6

Hunter Lot 5

Horse Area & Trails

Hunter Lot 1

Deer Run Trail

Old Village Trail

Hunter Lot 2

Kid's Fishing Pond

Group Tent

Hickory Hill Trailer Camp

Pine Grove Tent/Trailer

Oak Ridge Tent/Trailer

Hunter Lot 3

Hunter Lot 4

Red Oak Backpack Trail

Prairie Bluff Trail

TO 104

McKEE CREEK

Crabapple Backpack Area

TO BENVILLE

Legend	
SHOWERHOUSE	
RESTROOM	
PARKING	
HORSE TRAILS	
PARK OFFICE	
SHELTER	
DUMP STATION	
PICNIC AREA	
CONCESSION	
FISHING AREA	
HIKING TRAIL	— — —
FIRE LANE	▪▪▪▪▪

MAP

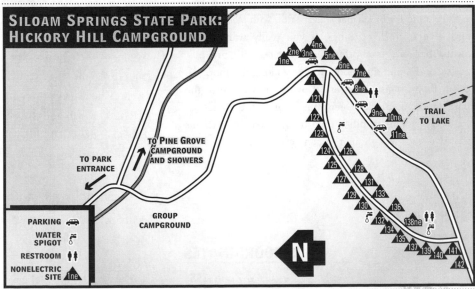

SILOAM SPRINGS STATE PARK: HICKORY HILL CAMPGROUND

TO PARK ENTRANCE

TO PINE GROVE CAMPGROUND AND SHOWERS

GROUP CAMPGROUND

TRAIL TO LAKE

1ne, 2ne, 3ne, 4ne, 5ne, 6ne, 7ne, 8ne, 9ne, 10ne, 11ne

H, 121, 122, 123, 124, 125, 126, 127, 128, 129, 130, 131, 132, 133, 134, 135, 136, 137, 138ne, 139, 140, 141, 142

Legend	
PARKING	
WATER SPIGOT	
RESTROOM	
NONELECTRIC SITE	1ne

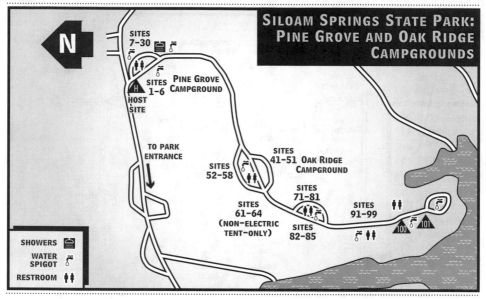

You can explore Siloam Springs' forested ridges via about 12 miles of hiking trails. The most challenging is the 4-mile Red Oak Backpack Trail, with steep slopes and several creek crossings. If you really want to get away, there are four primitive campsites with fire pits, tables, and a pit toilet, about midway along the loop. To camp there, register first and leave your vehicle at the park office, then take Deer Run Trail to the Red Oak trailhead, adding another mile to the hike. Avoid this trail when it's wet, though—it can get very muddy.

GPS COORDINATES

UTM Zone 15S
Easting 0674854
Northing 4418209
Latitude N 39° 53' 45.3490"
Longitude W 90° 57' 17.0599"

GETTING THERE

From Mount Sterling, take US 24 west about 10 miles to CR 2950 East, just before Clayton. Turn left, go 7 miles south to the three-way stop at Kellerville. Turn left onto CR 1200 North and drive 1.1 miles, then make a left on CR 2873 South and travel 2.4 miles south to the park entrance, on the left.

From Springfield, take I-72 west to Exit 35 (Griggsville). Head 11 miles north on IL 107 to IL 104, then take a left. Drive 12 miles to CR 2873 East, then hang a right and travel 5.8 miles to the park entrance, on the right.

15

JIM EDGAR PANTHER CREEK STATE FISH & WILDLIFE AREA

> *Camp in one of the unique three-sided wooden shelters and enjoy central Illinois' longest mountain-biking trail.*

JIM EDGAR PANTHER CREEK STATE Fish & Wildlife Area (JEPC) is one of Illinois' newest parks, and everything about it sparkles. The campgrounds are immaculate, the buildings clean and modern, and the trails well maintained. And JEPC is *big*—16,550 acres of rolling terrain—offering a beautiful mix of woods, prairie, lakes, and ponds, plenty to do, and camping options from the luxurious to the comfortably primitive.

Because JEPC covers such a huge area, there are various entrances, but the main one is from Ashland or Petersburg off Newmansville Road to the east. Go 1.4 miles from this entrance west to the office, turn left, and proceed less than 1 mile south to the main Prairie Lake Campground on the left. Stop here first to register with the campground host, where you can also purchase ice and firewood.

Go south from the main campground entrance to Wolf Road, where you'll see a sign for group and primitive camping. Turn left, then right, and go 0.2 miles to the walk-in camping parking lot. There are seven walk-in sites, spread along a well-mown grass trail, on the edge of the woods to the north. They're about 100 to 200 feet apart, and because of the way the trail curves you're mostly out of sight of your neighbors. Chances are you won't have many—this area doesn't always fill even on holiday weekends, and on an average fair weather weekend only two or three sites will be occupied.

Each site is equipped with a fire ring, table, trashcan, and, unique to JEPC in Illinois, a three-sided, roofed wooden shelter. Like everything else at JEPC, these look brand-new, sturdy, and attractive. They're about ten feet deep and provide protection from rain and sun, large enough that I've seen some campers simply stretch a tarp across the entrance and camp inside. My favorite is site 5—it's the most secluded, tucked back

RATINGS

Beauty: ✿ ✿ ✿ ✿
Privacy: ✿ ✿ ✿
Spaciousness: ✿ ✿ ✿ ✿
Quiet: ✿ ✿ ✿ ✿
Security: ✿ ✿ ✿ ✿ ✿
Cleanliness: ✿ ✿ ✿ ✿ ✿

into the woods—but the main criterion for choosing is how far you're willing to walk, from 0.1 mile for site 1 to less than 0.5 miles for site 7. The trail is smooth, and a wagon works well to transport your gear to the site. The vault toilets are located opposite site 3. You will need to get water at the group or main campground and can use the main shower house.

Either of the two group campgrounds, if not already taken or reserved, is available to individuals and family groups. They don't offer much shade, but there's lots of open space for pitching tents, plus water, restrooms, and a picnic shelter with electricity. Your "group" may be small, but you'll have to pay for a minimum of ten people. You can reserve one of these by phone for an additional $5.

The main campground doesn't offer much shade, either, but it is pretty, with spacious, flat, front-lawn kind of grassy expanses. All sites have electricity, but with a tent you'll want to avoid the expense of the 16 full-hookup sites. If you do want a bit of luxury, reserve one of the nine cabins well in advance. Each has two bunk beds, a double bed, a table, a ceiling fan, a heater, and electricity. You'll need to bring your own bedding. All are right on the lake, but cabins 8 and 9 are more secluded, with woods around.

JEPC offers plenty of recreational opportunities. Many come to fish, either in the 210-acre Prairie Lake (stocked with muskie, along with the usual panfish and catfish) or in one of the smaller, less busy lakes or ponds. Cyclists can enjoy the 9-mile paved biking loop trail, or the 24 miles of mountain-biking trail in two loops. With the gentle terrain at JEPC, the latter is fairly tame but scenic. It's open to bikers April 16 through October 31, and to hikers only during the rest of the year. For equestrians there is a 51-site campground and 26 miles of trails.

There is no concession at JEPC, but you can rent canoes from New Salem Canoes, which will deliver them anywhere in the park. They'll also give you basic canoeing instruction, and you can even arrange for guided trips around the lake or on the nearby Sangamon River. Check **www.newsalemcanoe.com** or call (217) 494-3957.

KEY INFORMATION

ADDRESS: 10149 County Highway 11, Chandlerville, IL

OPERATED BY: IDNR

CONTACT: (217) 452-7741, www.dnr.state.il.us/lands/land mgt/parks/r4/jepc.htm

OPEN: Year-round

SITES: Class D: 7 walk-in; Class A: 64 electric; Class AA: 18 full-hookups; 9 cabins

EACH SITE: Picnic table, fire ring; wooden shelter (Class D); electric (Class A & AA); sewer & water (Class AA)

ASSIGNMENT: First come, first served; cabins & group campground reservable

REGISTRATION: Register with campground host

FACILITIES: Water spigots, vault toilets, shower house

PARKING: At site (Class A & AA); in lot (Class D)

FEE: Class A: $20 per night, $30 per night holidays (add $5 for Class AA); Class D: $6 per night per tent (add $2 per night for shower use); cabin: $45 per night

ELEVATION: 599 feet

RESTRICTIONS: *Pets:* On leash only *Fires:* In fire rings only *Alcohol:* Not permitted in campgrounds *Vehicles:* 2 per site

MAP

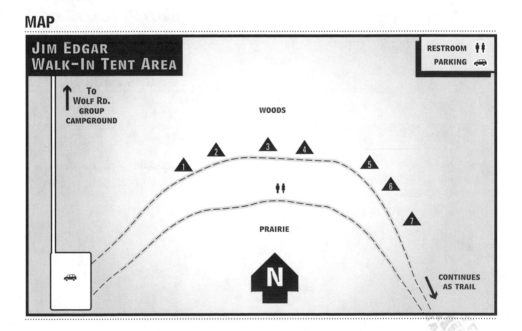

JIM EDGAR PRAIRIE LAKE CAMPGROUND

Legend:
- SHOWERS
- RESTROOM
- WATER ACCESS
- PLAYGROUND
- DUMP STATION
- WHEELCHAIR ACCESSIBLE
- BOAT DOCKS
- HOST SITE — H
- CABIN
- SHELTER

MAIN CAMP HOST

PRAIRIE LAKE

GROUP/ PRIMITIVE AREAS

N

MAP

JIM EDGAR WALK-IN TENT AREA

RESTROOM
PARKING

To WOLF RD. GROUP CAMPGROUND

WOODS

PRAIRIE

N

CONTINUES AS TRAIL

If you enjoy history, do not miss New Salem State Historic Site, south of nearby Petersburg. New Salem is a reconstruction of the village where Abraham Lincoln spent his early adulthood. You can tour the village homes, shops, museum, and visitor center, view demonstrations of daily life and work in the 1830s, and take in plays and concerts in the 250-seat outdoor theater. If you want to squeeze a bit of education into the kids' vacation, download any of the free activity guides available on the Web site. There is no admission cost, only a suggested donation. Call (217) 632-4000 or visit **www.lincolnsnewsalem.com** for more information. To get there from JEPC, go north 0.25 miles on Newmansville Road, follow it as it curves right and continues 11 miles into Petersburg (and becomes Douglas Street). Turn right on IL 123/97, and go 2.3 miles south to New Salem.

GETTING THERE

From Springfield, take I-72 west to Exit 76, then go north on IL 123. Go 11 miles to the T-intersection at IL 125 in Ashland. Turn left, go 2.8 miles to Newmansville Road, and turn right at the brown JEPC sign. Go 7 miles to the JEPC entrance on the left.

GPS COORDINATES

UTM Zone 15S
Easting 0752455
Northing 4431921
Latitude N 39° 59' 59.1679"
Longitude W 90° 2' 33.7232"

> *Friends Creek is a quiet park and campgroundt hat celebrates the prairies of central Illinois.*

FOLKS NOT FROM ILLINOIS (or from Chicago, which almost counts as a separate state) often think Illinois south of I-80 consists of nothing but mile after mile of flat corn and soybean fields. I hope the diversity of landscapes covered in this book serves to dispel that myth. However, around my hometown of Decatur in the center of the state, it's true. The glaciers scraped us smooth and left a rich layer of soil that defaults to luxurious prairie or, with a little coercion, supports vibrant agriculture.

Amid the fields and farms, Friends Creek Conservation Area is a park that celebrates the prairie. There are mature oak–hickory woods, to be sure, and its namesake creek winds through the area, but much of these 526 acres consists of beautiful open meadows and restored tallgrass prairie. The clean, quiet campground here is popular with locals but hardly known outside the area.

The campground consists of one large loop, with an avenue running down the middle. Most of the 17 electric sites are along the central road; the 19 non-electric sites are around the outer loop. Besides the fact that everything is clean and beautifully maintained (as are all the properties in the Macon County Conservation District), the sites are spacious, and many of the non-electric ones are canopied by tall, spreading oaks. The sites on the outside of the loop to the right as you enter—26, 29, 31, and 33—are my first choices for that reason. On the opposite side of the loop, sites are equally spacious but sunnier; sites 13 through 19 are good, with the best ones on the outside of the loop. Site 21, to the left as you enter, is also large and well shaded. If you want electricity, I recommend site 25, tucked into the trees at the southeast corner, or site 21. Those at the back are along a fence with farmland on the other side and aren't as attractive. You'll find water

RATINGS

Beauty: ✿ ✿ ✿ ✿
Privacy: ✿ ✿ ✿
Spaciousness: ✿ ✿ ✿
Quiet: ✿ ✿ ✿ ✿
Security: ✿ ✿ ✿ ✿ ✿
Cleanliness: ✿ ✿ ✿ ✿ ✿

spigots throughout the campground and an excellent shower building in the center. You can register with the campground host (at site 1) or at the self-registration board at the shower house.

You won't come to Friends Creek for solitude. On most weekends, all of the electric sites will be occupied by RVs, probably reserved well in advance. This is one of the few campgrounds I'm recommending where you may be just across the road from a trailer. However, the regulars who come to Friends Creek are a quiet bunch. You can usually walk in and get a good non-electric site, or you can reserve one in advance by credit card.

You can explore more of the woods and prairie around Friends Creek if you cross the highway to the parking area by the historic Bethel School. From there you can access two loop trails. As the name implies, the 2-mile Woodland Trail traverses woods before heading along Friends Creek. Sun Trail makes a 2.5-mile circuit through woods and across a gently sloping hillside meadow.

You can fish, but not swim, in Friends Creek. There is a superb 1,000-foot beach about 10 miles north at Clinton Lake, if you feel like taking a dip. It's usually busy on warm days, but there's plenty of room to spread out, and there are also changing rooms and showers. The large swimming area is marked by buoys and ranges from wading-pool shallow (for the little ones) to about six feet deep. The concession at the southern end sells sandwiches, snacks, and drinks. The beach is open Memorial Day to Labor Day, from 10 a.m. to 7 p.m., and the cost is $1 per person. Call (217) 935-8722 for more information. From Friends Creek, turn right out of the park onto Friends Creek Park Road and head 9.25 miles north until you cross the lake. Then take the first left into Clinton Lake State Park and follow the road and signs down to the beach.

If you want to do something more than lie in a hammock in the shade (which is a fine way to spend the day at Friends Creek), my favorite local place to hike is the Rock Springs Conservation Area, about 30 minutes away on the southwestern edge of Decatur. This is another Macon County Conservation District property, with 1,343 acres of woods and prairie. Here

KEY INFORMATION

ADDRESS: c/o Macon County Conservation District, 3939 Nearing Lane, Decatur, IL 62521

OPERATED BY: Macon County Conservation District

CONTACT: (217) 423-7708, www.macon county conservation.org/ friendscreek.php

OPEN: May 1–October 31

SITES: 19 non-electric, 17 electric

EACH SITE: Picnic table, fire ring

ASSIGNMENT: First come, first served; reservations available by phone with credit card

REGISTRATION: With campground host or at self-registration board

FACILITIES: Water spigots, vault toilets, shower house

PARKING: At site

FEE: Non-electric: $10 per night for county residents ($12 per night for non-residents); electric: $15 per night for county residents ($18 per night for non-residents)

ELEVATION: 679 feet

RESTRICTIONS: *Pets:* On leash only
Fires: In fire rings only
Alcohol: Not permitted
Vehicles: 2 per site
Other: 14-day limit; 1 RV or 2 tents per site; 6 people per site

MAP

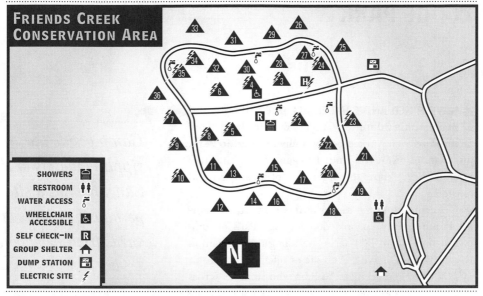

FRIENDS CREEK CONSERVATION AREA

SHOWERS
RESTROOM
WATER ACCESS
WHEELCHAIR ACCESSIBLE
SELF CHECK-IN
GROUP SHELTER
DUMP STATION
ELECTRIC SITE

N

GETTING THERE

From I-72 at Exit 156, go north 0.7 miles on IL 48 to Duroc Road. Turn left and go 1 mile to Friends Creek Park Road. Turn right and drive 0.25 miles to the park entrance, on the right.

GPS COORDINATES

UTM Zone 16T
Easting 0347826
Northing 4432599
Latitude N 40° 1' 47.6201"
Longitude W 88° 47' 0.4741"

you can hike up some actual hills (albeit small ones) along the 9 miles of interconnected trails that traverse the area. As well, there is a 2.5-mile paved bike trail. My favorite hike is the 2.5-mile River Trail that follows the Sangamon River (the lower portions may be flooded or muddy in the spring). Trail maps are available at Friends Creek. Don't miss the nature center, which has live fish and reptiles, a bird-watching window, and excellent interactive exhibits that kids will enjoy. To get to Rock Springs from Friends Creek, take I-72 west toward Decatur to Exit 133, which puts you on US 36 East. Go to the stoplight and turn right onto Wyckles Road. Drive 2.1 miles to Rock Springs Road, turn left, go 1 mile to Brozio Lane, and then head 0.5 miles to the entrance, on the left.

17
LODGE PARK

I HAVE HIKED AND CAMPED ALL OVER Illinois, and lived within 30 miles of Lodge Park for half of my life. I've even worked occasionally at Allerton Park, just 8 miles away. Yet until I began researching this book, I didn't know this little gem of a campground existed.

According to the ranger at this Piatt County Forest Preserve, most people don't. Lodge Park encompasses only about 500 acres straddling the Sangamon River. It doesn't have a Web site or offer a brochure or even a campground map. Visitors who stumble across it are often just as pleasantly surprised as I was. Lodge Park offers the chance to camp right beside the rippling waters of the Sangamon at a site perhaps hundreds of yards from the nearest neighbor. You can do a little fishing and hiking, but you'll come here for a tranquil stay with few neighbors, leaving you with fields, woods, and water almost to yourself.

The ranger will tell you Lodge Park offers "roughly 20" campsites. The uncertainty is due to the fact that much of the campground is open field, and campers can set up anywhere within that area. The more or less official sites, unnumbered, are wherever you see a picnic table and fire ring—I counted 13. The camping area consists of a large loop, about 1.5 miles around, with a single road bisecting the loop from the entrance.

Drive around the southern part of the loop, and you'll find other sites scattered in a grassy field, some with large trees, and most close to water and restrooms. Those south of the road across are spacious but closer together; those just north of it are farther apart. For the best site in this area, take the entrance road straight across the field and turn right. Away from the road, this site affords a great view of the Sangamon and has some wooded cover.

The star campsites for privacy are the four in the mixed pine and deciduous forest at the northern end. For these you'll have to park roadside and walk a bit, at

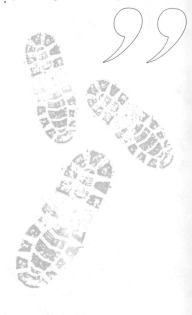

Camp beside the rippling waters of the Sangamon at a site perhaps hundreds of yards from neighbors.

RATINGS

Beauty: ✿ ✿ ✿
Privacy: ✿ ✿ ✿ ✿
Spaciousness: ✿ ✿ ✿ ✿ ✿
Quiet: ✿ ✿ ✿ ✿
Security: ✿ ✿ ✿ ✿
Cleanliness: ✿ ✿ ✿ ✿

ADDRESS: 1852 North Old Route 47, Monticello, IL 61856

OPERATED BY: Piatt County Forest Preserve District

CONTACT: (217) 762-4531, www.monticello tourism.org/ parks_rec.php

OPEN: Year-round (but closed to vehicles Apr. 1–Dec. 1)

SITES: About 13

EACH SITE: Picnic table, grill, fire ring

ASSIGNMENT: First come, first served

REGISTRATION: Set up and park staff will come by or register at office

FACILITIES: Water spigots, vault toilets

PARKING: At campsite or off road nearby

FEE: $5 per night

ELEVATION: 663 feet

RESTRICTIONS: *Pets:* On leash only
Fires: In fire rings only
Alcohol: Not permitted
Vehicles: 2 per site
Other: 14-day limit; 3 tents, or 1 RV and 1 tent per site

most 100 feet. The reward is a sense of isolation rarely found at any established campground.

Head north, counterclockwise around the loop, and watch for a trail into the woods. This will lead you to the first wooded site, hidden from the road. The next, at the northernmost point, is right on the Sangamon River. It was muddy when I visited because it had recently rained; it can flood when the river is high. The next two, in the northwest corner of the campground, are my favorites. The one on the east is larger and overlooks the river, while the one to the west is well away from the road—watch for the trail, or you'll drive right past it.

Reservations are not accepted, but Lodge Park is rarely full, even on the Memorial Day or Labor Day weekends. The only exception is around the Fourth of July, when the park is packed with campers and is the site of Monticello's fireworks display. Don't come looking for peace and quiet from about June 20 to July 5! Occasionally, scout or youth groups camp here as well, but they usually give notice, so you can call ahead to see if you'd be sharing the grounds with a large group.

Lodge Park is open for camping year-round. However, it is closed to vehicular traffic from December 1 to April 1. You can park at the entrance and walk in, but you'll have to carry your gear. Also, note that the park is down the road from a small subdivision, so you may see some locals jogging or walking dogs.

When water levels are low enough (usually in the summer), you can also cross the Sangamon on foot via the concrete ford in the southwest corner of the campground. There are about 150 wooded acres with clearly marked trails on the other side. If you don't mind getting your feet wet, you can sometimes camp over there—check with the ranger for permission.

From Lodge Park you can also visit nearby Allerton Park, voted one of the "seven wonders of Illinois" by state residents. Allerton was the estate of the gentleman farmer and art collector Robert Allerton, who devoted three decades to developing the ornamental gardens surrounding his manor house. Today the University of Illinois manages the park for recreation, education, and research purposes. You can hike more than

MAP

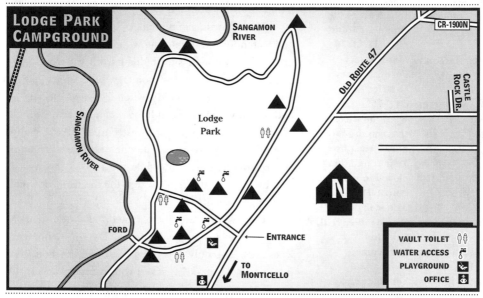

LODGE PARK CAMPGROUND

SANGAMON RIVER

CR-1900N

OLD ROUTE 47

CASTLE ROCK DR.

SANGAMON RIVER

Lodge Park

FORD

← ENTRANCE

TO MONTICELLO

VAULT TOILET
WATER ACCESS
PLAYGROUND
OFFICE

N

14 miles of well-marked trails through the gardens, unique statuary, and natural areas adjacent to the Sangamon River.

Allerton is open from 8 a.m. to dusk. The manor house itself now serves as a conference center and is usually not open to the public. For trail maps and more information, stop by the visitor center, or visit **www .allerton.uiuc.edu.**

From Lodge Park: Turn right onto Old State Road 47 and drive to I-72 West. Proceed 2 miles to Exit 164, and turn left onto Bridge Street. Drive 0.5 miles, turn right onto Old SR 47, and go 2 miles to CR 625 East. Turn left, go 1 mile to the T-intersection, turn right, and drive 0.5 miles to the entrance to Allerton, on the left.

GETTING THERE

From Decatur, take I-72 East to Exit 166, turn right, then make the next right onto Old Route 47. Drive 0.5 miles north to the park entrance, on the left. From Champaign, take I-72 West to Exit 169 and turn right onto Old Route 47. Go 2.5 miles north to the park entrance, on the right.

GPS COORDINATES

UTM Zone 16T
Easting 0366742
Northing 4435903
Latitude N 40° 03' 46.28"
Longitude W 88° 33' 45.11"

The Middle Fork of the Vermilion River is Illinois' only Wild and Scenic River, with clear waters, rocky bluffs, and steep banks.

THE TRAILS AND CAMPGROUNDS at Middle Fork State Fish & Wildlife Area are used primarily by equestrians, but don't let that scare you away. The two times I've been there I've seen few riders, none of whom were camping, and the only evidence I saw (or smelled) that horses had been there was in the parking lot by the campground. There's one little-used section of the campground that's just for tent campers, plus secluded hike-in sites that most visitors never see. If you don't mind going without a shower, this is a quiet alternative to the busier nearby Kickapoo State Park.

The campsites with vehicular access are in the southern part of Middle Fork. From the park gate on CR 2250 North, go 0.75 miles to the parking lot after the road turns left. As long as the road to the campsites isn't too muddy for vehicles, the gate at the north end of the lot will be open, and you can drive through. There are four camps along the road, each with multiple sites. Camps A, C, and D are for equestrians only, and on an average weekend you may find half those sites occupied. Camp B, however, is just for tent campers. It has four spacious, grassy sites that are well separated and shaded by towering oaks; each site has a table and fire ring. The farthest site is about 225 feet from the road, but all are good. Some weekends it's completely empty, and others you may have a neighbor or two. You'll find water and toilets nearby at Camp C, or at the north end of the parking lot.

If you really want to get away, and don't mind working for it, Middle Fork also has seven backpacking sites around a pond in the woods, accessed from the northern part of the park. From CR 900 East, turn right onto CR 2400 North. Go about 0.4 miles, just past the ranger station, to the parking area on the right. If you plan to camp, call the office at Kickapoo State Park first, and leave a note on your dashboard. The 1-mile

RATINGS

Beauty: ☆ ☆ ☆
Privacy: ☆ ☆ ☆ ☆
Spaciousness: ☆ ☆ ☆
Quiet: ☆ ☆ ☆ ☆ ☆
Security: ☆ ☆ ☆ ☆
Cleanliness: ☆ ☆ ☆ ☆

trail to the pond begins in the east or left corner of the parking lot. Proceed straight ahead across a field to the edge of the woods. From here you need to look for the continuation of the trail into the woods, since it's not marked. You cross an old road at about 0.5 miles. A GPS or compass is helpful—the pond campsites are about 1 mile south-by-southeast (160°) from the parking area, at North 40° 12' 18.08", West 87° 45' 18.08", and the trail is fairly direct. If you make it (and I did, unfortunately with about 0.5 miles of unnecessary extra steps—hence the GPS recommendation), the reward is absolute seclusion in a beautiful spot. There's no potable water, but each site has a fire ring and a table; there's a pit toilet near the signboard and self-registration post. The seven sites are well separated, but that's hardly important because you will almost certainly be the only person camping there.

The Middle Fork of the Vermilion River forms the eastern border of the Fish & Wildlife Area. This is Illinois' only nationally designed Wild and Scenic River, with sparkling clear waters, rocky bluffs, and steep banks devoid of development. There are two canoe-access points, one at Kinney's Ford, north of the ranger station, off 2600 North Road, and the second at Bunker Hill, at the end of the campground road. If you want to rent canoes, head to Kickapoo Landing in Kickapoo State Park, 4 miles south of Middle Fork. They'll shuttle you and the canoe back up to Middle Fork, and you canoe down to their place at Kickapoo at your own pace—then you can end the day with dinner at their Dockside Café. They offer an 8-mile trip from Bunker Hill, and an 11-mile trip from Kinney's Ford. Call (217) 446-8399 for reservations on the weekends, and check **www.kicka poolanding.com** for more information.

The opposite bank of the river is Kennekuk County Park of the Vermilion County Conservation District, which has its own set of natural and historic attractions. Here you can hike 10 miles of trails that traverse woodland, wetland, prairie, and riverine ecosystems, as well as the 7.5-mile trail around Lake Mingo, all limited to hikers only. Lake Mingo offers boating and fishing and has a concession where you can rent johnboats, canoes, and pedal boats. The visitor

KEY INFORMATION

ADDRESS: c/o Kickapoo State Park, 10906 Kickapoo Park Rd., Oakwood, IL

OPERATED BY: IDNR

CONTACT: (217) 442-4915, www.dnr.state.il. us/lands/land mgt/parks/r3/ middle.htm

OPEN: Around April 1– Nov. 1

SITES: Class C: 4 tent sites, Class C: 24 equestrian sites, 7 hike-in sites

EACH SITE: Picnic table, fire ring

ASSIGNMENT: First come, first served

REGISTRATION: Set up and park staff will come by; for hike-in sites, call in advance and self-register at site

FACILITIES: Vault toilets; water spigots (campground only)

PARKING: At site (campground sites); at trailhead (hike-in sites)

FEE: $8 per night (campground); $6 per night (hike-in)

ELEVATION: 668 feet

RESTRICTIONS: *Pets:* On leash only *Fires:* In fire rings only *Alcohol:* Permitted *Vehicles:* 2 per site *Other:* 14-day limit; 2 tents per site; 4 adults or 1 family per site

MAP

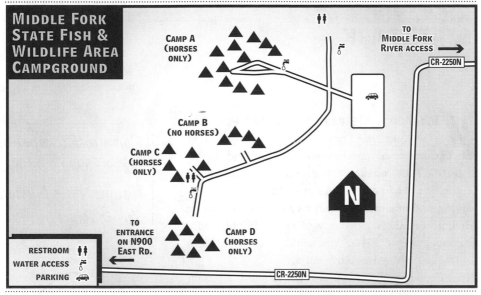

MIDDLE FORK STATE FISH & WILDLIFE AREA CAMPGROUND

CAMP A (HORSES ONLY)

TO MIDDLE FORK RIVER ACCESS →

CR-2250N

CAMP B (NO HORSES)

CAMP C (HORSES ONLY)

N

TO ENTRANCE ON N900 EAST RD.

CAMP D (HORSES ONLY)

RESTROOM
WATER ACCESS
PARKING

CR-2250N

GETTING THERE

From I-74, take Exit 206 north onto Newtown Road (CR 900 North). Go 5 miles, turn right at the park sign onto CR 2250 North, and drive 0.9 miles to the southern park gate.

GPS COORDINATES

UTM Zone 16T
Easting 0435908
Northing 4449836
Latitude N 40° 11' 47.3092"
Longitude W 87° 45' 10.8108"

center is great for maps and brochures, but don't miss the natural history museum and 1,000-gallon aquarium inside. History buffs will enjoy walking through Bunker Hill historic area, with its restored chapel, school, print shop, barbershop, and train depot, among other buildings, open summer Saturdays from 1 to 4 p.m. For more information, check **www.vccd.org/gikennekuk.html.** To get to Kennekuk from Middle Fork, go north on CR 900 East to CR 2600 North. Turn right and drive 3.3 miles east to Henning Road (CR 1). Turn right and continue 3.3 miles south to the Kennekuk entrance, on the right.

19

KICKAPOO STATE PARK

KICKAPOO STATE PARK IS A GREAT PLACE to play. Sure, the campsites are spacious, tent campers can use the shower house, and there's a terrific little restaurant, but the prime attraction is recreation. The park offers scenic (and even rugged) hiking and mountain biking, excellent fishing, scuba diving, and the opportunity to canoe Illinois' only National Scenic River. You could come here for a quiet, do-nothing weekend—but why?

Kickapoo owes its diverse recreation and terrain to the fact that these lands were once open strip mines. The state of Illinois purchased them in 1939, and over the years nature has transformed them into deep, clear ponds, steep hills, and wooded ravines. Twenty-two ponds and lakes cover more than 220 of Kickapoo's 2,842 acres, providing ample space for lots to do.

As you enter the park from the east, go about 0.25 miles past the bridge to the entrance to Brian Plawer Campground on the right. Pass the check-in station, take the first right turn, and go down the hill to the Erie loop of the campground. As you enter the loop, you'll see the sign for the tent-camping area on the left. On the right is the grassy clearing where you can park after you've unloaded your gear.

The 18 walk-in tent sites, numbers 119 through 102 (in that order from the parking lot) extend along a 0.25-mile footpath that parallels a ridge overlooking the lake below. All are sufficiently spacious, with a picnic table and ground grill. Vault toilets are behind site 110, and water spigots available in the campground loops at either end of the tent area. There isn't much brush between you and your neighbors, but sites 106 and 109 are set back the farthest from the trail and offer the most space. On an average non-holiday weekend, this area is about half full, so you should be able to find something suitable.

> *Come to Kickapoo for the chance to canoe Illinois' only National Scenic River.*

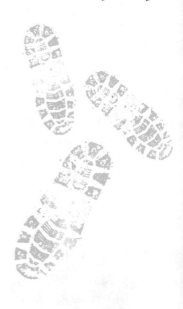

RATINGS

Beauty: ✯ ✯ ✯ ✯
Privacy: ✯ ✯ ✯
Spaciousness: ✯ ✯ ✯
Quiet: ✯ ✯ ✯ ✯
Security: ✯ ✯ ✯ ✯
Cleanliness: ✯ ✯ ✯ ✯

KEY INFORMATION

ADDRESS: 10906 Kickapoo Park Road, Oakwood, IL 61858

OPERATED BY: IDNR

CONTACT: (217) 442-4915, www.dnr.state.il.us/lands/landmgt/parks/r3/kickapoo.htm

OPEN: Year-round

SITES: Class C: 18 walk-in tent sites; Class B: 64 non-electric sites; Class A: 100 electric sites

EACH SITE: Electric (Class A only); picnic table, fire ring

ASSIGNMENT: First come, first served

REGISTRATION: Set up first, then register at office

FACILITIES: Water spigots, vault toilets, showers (may be closed in winter)

PARKING: At site (Class A & B); in lot (Class C)

FEE: Class A: $20 per night, $30 per night holidays; Class B: $10 per night; Class C: $8 per night; $2 less when showers are closed

ELEVATION: 559 feet

RESTRICTIONS: *Pets:* On leash only
Fires: In fire rings only
Alcohol: Permitted
Vehicles: 2 per site
Other: 14-day limit; 1 RV and 1 tent, or 2 tents per site; 4 adults or 1 family per site

Besides the walk-in sites, many of the drive-in sites are surprisingly large, with plenty of flat grassy space for pitching tents. If you'd prefer a drive-in site, it's generally best to go for one of the smaller loops, such as Fox, with 15 electric sites, or Erie, with 33 non-electric sites, and try for those on the outside of the loop. In Erie, if you need two adjacent sites, I recommend 132 and 133, 148 and 149, or 150 and 152. For a single site, I really like 129, which is spacious and right by the stairs down to the large fishing dock on Long Lake. In Fox, site 90 is nice; 95 is my favorite, with a beautiful view of the lake below.

The Illini and Miami loops of the campground offer more-typical RV sites and would be my last choice for tent camping. If you are stuck there, try for sites 74 through 81 on the east side of Illini—they're a bit bigger and back up to woods.

Kickapoo has a secondary campground—Redear Campground—0.5 miles south of the intersection past the bridge at the park entrance. It has 30 non-electric sites, water, and vault toilets, and campers can use the showers in Plawer Campground. I don't think its sites are nearly as attractive as the good sites in the main campground.

In my opinion, Kickapoo State Park can also boast one of the nicest, friendliest, and best-run park concessions in Illinois. Kickapoo Landing is located just past the bridge into the park. They offer 8- or 13-mile canoe or kayak trips and 2-mile tube trips on the Middle Fork of the Vermilion River, or you can rent a canoe, kayak, double kayak, or paddleboat by the hour, half day, or day to explore Clear Lake and Inland Sea in the park. The best part is that they shuttle you upstream and you head back to Kickapoo Landing—no need to wait on or hurry to meet a bus at your take-out point. You can even check your keys at the boathouse, so you don't risk losing them in the river. They also sell bait, fishing supplies, ice, and firewood. Check the Web site, **www.kickapoo.landing.com,** for current information. On weekends call in advance to reserve a boat, and on weekdays call to schedule a shuttle time: (217) 446-8399.

Kickapoo Landing also runs Dockside Café, open daily for breakfast, lunch, and dinner from Memorial

MAP

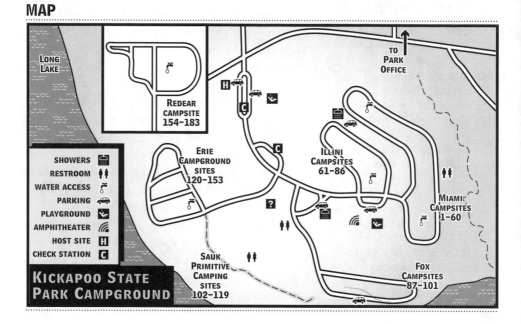

KICKAPOO STATE PARK CAMPGROUND

SHOWERS
RESTROOM
WATER ACCESS
PARKING
PLAYGROUND
AMPHITHEATER
HOST SITE **H**
CHECK STATION **C**

LONG LAKE

REDEAR CAMPSITE 154–183

ERIE CAMPGROUND SITES 120–153

ILLINI CAMPSITES 61–86

MIAMI CAMPSITES 1–60

SAUK PRIMITIVE CAMPING SITES 102–119

FOX CAMPSITES 87–101

TO PARK OFFICE

Day to Labor Day, and on the weekends in the fall and spring. You can enjoy live music there on Friday and Tuesday evenings during the summer.

Kickapoo is one of the few parks in Illinois that allows scuba diving. If you register and show proper certification, you can dive in Sportsman's Lake or Inland Sea. Don't expect crystal-clear waters—visibility is usually ten feet or less—but it's worth trying if you enjoy diving.

There are also more than 10 miles of mountain-biking trails of varying degrees of difficulty in the northern part of the park. The local Kickapoo Mountain Bike Club maintains these trails, and you can find trail maps and descriptions, as well as recent conditions, on their Web site, **www.kickapoombc.org.**

GETTING THERE

From I-74, take Exit 206 north onto Newtown Road. Go 1 mile, turn right at the park sign onto CR 1880 North, then go 2 miles to the park entrance.

GPS COORDINATES

UTM Zone 16T
Easting 0436261
Northing 4443285
Latitude N 40° 8' 14.9379"
Longitude W 87° 44' 53.5751"

20
FOREST GLEN COUNTY PRESERVE

> *Don't miss the stunning view of the Vermilion River valley from the top of the 72-foot observation tower.*

I KNEW THAT FOREST GLEN COUNTY PRESERVE was another underappreciated gem when a staff member told me they often get visitors from Danville—14 miles away—who are surprised to discover this beautiful spot virtually in their own backyard. Forest Glen *is* a surprise. On the drive there, you'd swear there's nothing but cornfields, until you stumble across this enclave of 1,800 acres of wooded ravines and tallgrass prairie adjacent to the Vermilion River. The well-maintained grounds, facilities, and hiking trails, along with a variety of interpretive programs, make it easy to enjoy this diverse bit of west-central Illinois.

Forest Glen also does tent camping right—there's a separate campground for tent campers that's walk-in only and is just far enough from parking to keep vehicle noise to a minimum but not too far to carry your gear. And all campers get to use the showers in the main campground—pretty close to ideal for me.

As you enter the preserve, go straight, then turn right at the campground sign. You'll first pass the ranger station, where you'll return to register after you've set up camp—they're open Monday through Thursday, 5 to 6 p.m., and Friday through Sunday noon to 8 p.m. The next right leads to the walk-in tent area. You can unload your vehicle in the circular lot at the end of the road and then park in the lot just before it.

The walk-in tent-camping area consists of a loop with 14 sites, all wooded and well shaded, each with a table and fire ring. Generally, the sites on the outside of the loop are larger and farther apart, and most look out over the wooded ravine and small creek that encircles this little hill. Sites 1, 2, 5, 7, and 13 are a bit small, but sites 3, 4, 6, and 12 are more spacious. Sites 8, 9, 10, and 11 are clustered together—any one of these would be fine if the others weren't occupied. Site 14 is my first choice—it's set apart from the others yet still close to

RATINGS

Beauty: ✪ ✪ ✪ ✪
Privacy: ✪ ✪ ✪
Spaciousness: ✪ ✪ ✪
Quiet: ✪ ✪ ✪ ✪
Security: ✪ ✪ ✪ ✪ ✪
Cleanliness: ✪ ✪ ✪ ✪ ✪

parking. No site is far, though—you won't walk more than 200 feet to get to any of them. There is a water spigot and vault toilets beside the loop entrance. On an average fair-weather weekend, you can expect this campground to be half full.

Instead of turning right toward the walk-in campground, continue straight and you'll end up at the family campground. These 42 sites all have gravel pull-ins, a table, and a large fire ring, and they offer plenty of grass-covered space for pitching a tent. Pass the campground host and shower house and turn right to reach the eight non-electric sites on the south side of the road—29, 30, 33, 34, 37, 38, 41, and 42. These are large sites, though not as well shaded as those in the walk-in campground. Willow Creek Pond sits behind them, and there's a small fishing dock by site 33. The campground host also sells firewood and ice.

Backpackers can camp for free at one of two places along the 11-mile River Ridge loop trail, at the 3-mile and 7.5-mile points. You must register in advance, preferably at least a week. The registration form is available on the Web site and can be emailed or faxed in. The trail begins at the staff office parking lot, where you can also pick up a detailed trail map.

If you have a head for heights and your legs can stand the climb, you shouldn't miss the view from the top of the 72-foot observation tower. As you're entering the park, take the second right, following the signs to the observation-tower parking. The hike is 0.2 miles down a wide gravel path along a ridge with wooded valleys on either side. Most old fire towers around the state have either been torn down or locked up over liability concerns, but this one is open from dawn to dusk, and each level is reassuringly surrounded by chain-link fence. (You should still hang on to smaller children when ascending.) Enjoy the stunning view of the Vermilion River valley before descending to hike 0.15 miles down to the Vermilion itself. Here you can connect with other well-marked trails, ranging from easy to rugged. Pick up a trail guide and map at the staff office.

On weekends Forest Glen offers a variety of activities that families with kids will particularly appreciate. North of the campgrounds, check out the Sycamore

KEY INFORMATION

ADDRESS:	20301 East 900 North Road, Westville, IL
OPERATED BY:	Vermilion County Conservation District
CONTACT:	(217) 662-2142, www.vccd.org/giforestglen.html
OPEN:	Year-round
SITES:	14 walk-in tent sites, 34 electric sites, 8 non-electric sites, 2 backpacking areas
EACH SITE:	Picnic table, fire ring
ASSIGNMENT:	First come, first served
REGISTRATION:	Set up, then register at ranger station; backpackers register in advance
FACILITIES:	Water spigots, vault toilets, shower house
PARKING:	In lot (walk-in sites); at site
FEE:	Non-electric & walk-in sites: $10 per night; electric sites: $15 per night; backpacking sites: free
ELEVATION:	640 feet
RESTRICTIONS:	*Pets:* On leash only *Fires:* In fire rings only *Alcohol:* Permitted *Vehicles:* 2 per site *Other:* 14-day limit; 1 RV and 1 tent, or 2 tents per site; no collecting of firewood

MAP

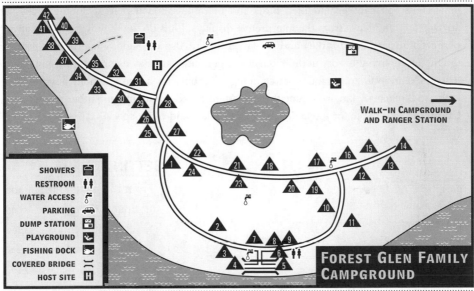

SHOWERS
RESTROOM
WATER ACCESS
PARKING
DUMP STATION
PLAYGROUND
FISHING DOCK
COVERED BRIDGE
HOST SITE

WALK-IN CAMPGROUND
AND RANGER STATION

FOREST GLEN FAMILY
CAMPGROUND

MAP

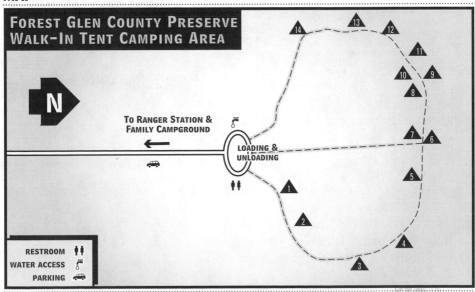

FOREST GLEN COUNTY PRESERVE
WALK-IN TENT CAMPING AREA

N

TO RANGER STATION &
FAMILY CAMPGROUND

LOADING &
UNLOADING

RESTROOM
WATER ACCESS
PARKING

Valley Nature Center, open on Sundays from Memorial Day to Labor Day from 1 to 4 p.m. Here you can see mounted birds and mammals, touch pelts, examine rocks and arrowheads, and learn from the interpretive displays. Outside the building you can always observe the caged wild turkey and red-tailed hawk. Also on Sunday afternoons, head up the hill to see living history at the Pioneer Homestead. Saturday evenings from June to the first weekend in October, join your camping neighbors for a free one-hour hayride. Meet at the staff office—7 p.m. from June through August, and 6 p.m. in September and October. Check the staff office for a schedule of guided hikes and other special activities.

GETTING THERE

From I-74, take Exit 215 and follow Georgetown Road (US 150) south 4.2 miles. Turn left on Main Street at the CVS pharmacy and follow the road 7.3 miles to the park entrance, on the left.

GPS COORDINATES

UTM Zone 16T
Easting 0452586
Northing 4427910
Latitude N 40° 0' 0.1635"
Longitude W 87° 33' 19.6486"

> *You'llp robably have this little camping area all to yourself.*

CALHOUN COUNTY IN WESTERN ILLINOIS is almost an island—35 miles long and barely 6 miles wide for most of its length, it's a hilly, heavily wooded peninsula tucked between the Illinois and Mississippi rivers. To get there from the east, west, or south requires using the single bridge or one of three ferries. Visitors can discover small towns, secluded wild places, and even archeological excavations that reveal 8,000 years of human habitation. And amid this is one quiet place to tent camp: the McCully Heritage Project.

McCully is a private nonprofit foundation, the legacy of Howard and Eva McCully, established to promote environmental education and enjoyment of the natural, cultural, and historical resources of the lower Illinois River valley. Today the foundation manages these 940 acres for a variety of programs, including limited primitive camping.

I have described some campgrounds as "underappreciated" or "less frequented"; McCully could be called "virtually unknown," at least in terms of camping. Camping has been available there only since 2006; so far they have averaged about five camping parties per year, almost all from nearby counties.

When you arrive at McCully, park in the lot in front of the pavilion. Walk left, past the white house that serves as the office and visitor center, and behind the red barn you'll see a signboard directing you to the campsites. Put your donation in one of the envelopes and slip it into the red box.

The three campsites are northwest of the barn and surrounded by woods. Site 1, to the left, has the most shade. Sites 2 and 3 share a large, open, grassy area to the right; site 3 is a bit shadier than 2. You'll find a picnic table and fire ring, and probably some firewood neatly stacked there for your use—if not, help yourself

RATINGS

Beauty: ✪ ✪ ✪ ✪
Privacy: ✪ ✪ ✪ ✪ ✪
Spaciousness: ✪ ✪ ✪ ✪ ✪
Quiet: ✪ ✪ ✪ ✪ ✪
Security: ✪ ✪ ✪ ✪
Cleanliness: ✪ ✪ ✪ ✪

to the pile under the pine tree behind the barn. Pit toilets are in the white building by the barn, and water pumps by the pavilion and in the yard behind the office. There's nothing spectacular in terms of scenery or even isolation—you're still fairly close to the road and the house where the groundskeeper lives—just simple campsites, and probably no one else camping. Though not required, I suggest calling ahead if you want to camp—there's always the possibility a school group has scheduled a field trip the very day you want to come. Although there are just three sites now, if demand should increase they may add more.

McCully's 940 acres offer plenty of places to explore. Go north past the campsites to see the historic 19th-century log cabin. Just beyond that are two ponds where you can fish or just watch turtles sunning themselves. South of the road is a boardwalk trail through a wetland. Beyond this is about 15 miles of secluded hiking trails, mostly wooded, with abundant wildlife and scenic overlooks of the Illinois River valley. You will have to work a bit to enjoy it—the entrance to McCully lies in a valley, and everything to the north and south is uphill. But the rewards are well worth it. You may see some of the myriad bird species that have been sighted there, as well as deer, wild turkey, fox, coyote, and even the elusive and endangered bobcat. From the southernmost overlook, you can see 21 miles downriver to Pere Marquette Park. The 12 miles of trails to the south are the most extensive, and a trail map is necessary—they should be at the main kiosk by the parking lot and will eventually be online. However, both the trails and the map are a work-in-progress, so check before you go. Note that the southern trails may be shared with equestrians from April 15 to October 1.

For backpackers, there are also two hike-in campsites in the southern section, each less than 1 mile (uphill!) from the wetland parking area. There are no facilities, just a clearing in the woods, but it's certainly peaceful. Or you can rent a rustic house with electricity, water, and vehicular access. Call for more information.

If you think archeology means pyramids and ancient Egypt, check out the Center for American Archeology in Kampsville, on IL 100 just south of the

KEY INFORMATION

ADDRESS:	P.O. Box 244, Kampsville, IL 62053
OPERATED BY:	McCully Heritage Foundation
CONTACT:	(618) 653-4687, www.mccully heritage.org
OPEN:	Year-round
SITES:	3 primitive walk-in sites, 2 hike-in sites
EACH SITE:	Picnic table and fire ring (walk-in sites only)
ASSIGNMENT:	First come, first served
REGISTRATION:	Self-registration kiosk
FACILITIES:	Water spigots, vault toilets
PARKING:	At lot
FEE:	$7.50 per night suggested donation; $5 donation requested for firewood
ELEVATION:	457 feet
RESTRICTIONS:	*Pets:* On leash only *Fires:* In fire rings only *Alcohol:* Not permitted *Vehicles:* 2 per site *Other:* No cutting or gathering of firewood

MAP

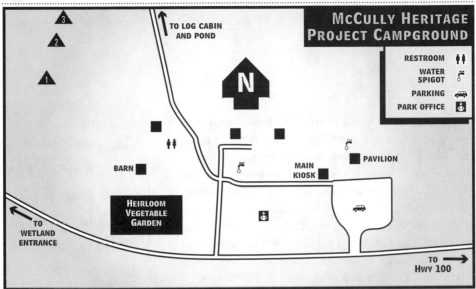

McCULLY HERITAGE PROJECT CAMPGROUND

TO LOG CABIN AND POND

RESTROOM	
WATER SPIGOT	
PARKING	
PARK OFFICE	

BARN

PAVILION

MAIN KIOSK

HEIRLOOM VEGETABLE GARDEN

TO WETLAND ENTRANCE

TO HWY 100

GETTING THERE

Follow IL 108 West to the Illinois River (54 miles from I-55, Exit 60; 22 miles from US 67). Take the free ferry (which runs 24 hours) across the river to Kampsville, then turn left onto IL 100. Go 1.1 miles south to Crawford Creek Road, turn right, and go 0.5 miles to the entrance, on the right.

GPS COORDINATES

UTM Zone 15T
Easting 0705137
Northing 4350802
Latitude N 39° 16' 56.3203"
Longitude W 90° 37' 17.8957"

ferry crossing. This fascinating museum focuses on the prehistory of the area around the confluence of the Illinois and Mississippi rivers, which has been called the "Nile of North America" for the sophisticated Native American settlements that developed there as far back as 6000 B.C. If you have more time, you can visit a working archeological dig during the summer and even participate. The museum is open May through October, Tuesday to Sunday. Admission is free, but donations are appreciated. Check their Web site, **www .caa-archeology.org,** or call (618) 653-4316 for information on special programs.

McCully is just 25 miles north of the much better known (and much busier) Pere Marquette State Park, popular for its scenic trails and rustic Civilian Conservation Corps–built lodge. However, that campground is nearly always full—camp at McCully, drive down for the day, and have dinner in the excellent lodge dining room. To get there, take IL 100 south almost 25 miles to the park entrance, on the left. For more information on area attractions, check **www.greatriverroad.com.**

AS I DROVE AROUND THE BEND from the entrance of Beaver Dam State Park to the lakefront, I immediately wanted to stop, get out of the car, and stretch out on one of the benches facing the lake to take in the view. The lake is the centerpiece of this picturesque park, with its gently rolling hills, mature oak and hickory woods, marshlands, and picnic areas overlooking the lake. The man-made parts—lakefront, restaurant, pavilions, docks, and restrooms—are also well maintained and attractive.

Visit just about any weekend during camping season, and you'll see that Beaver Dam is a popular destination. The campground fills up most weekends from mid-April to the end of October by Friday afternoon. If solitude is what you want, Beaver Dam is probably not your first choice, at least Friday to Sunday. However, if you're looking for a comfortable, secure, and scenic place for the whole family to camp, fish, and enjoy the outdoors together, and you have the luxury of coming before Friday, Beaver Dam is a good choice.

Though reservations are not accepted, Beaver Dam is one of the few state parks where you can set up a tent or RV in advance to reserve your site. Regular campers seem willing to pay for the extra nights to get their pick of sites.

So if you're bringing the whole clan, grandma and grandpa can park their RV on Thursday at one of the 66 electric sites and put up tents to claim the sites you'll want on Friday. You and the kids can rough it in the tents, and those who want a real bed can reserve (well in advance) the cabin right next to the modern shower house. You'll all be within an easy walk of one another. Fish in the morning and teach the kids to clean their catch at the excellent fish-cleaning station by the boat launch. Rent a boat with an electric motor for an afternoon excursion on the 59-acre lake, or hike one of the

> *This scenic little park is a comfortable and secure place for the whole family to camp, fish, and enjoy the outdoors together.*

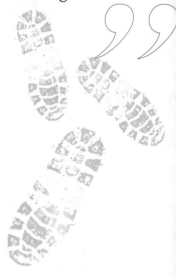

RATINGS

Beauty: ✵ ✵ ✵ ✵ ✵
Privacy: ✵ ✵ ✵
Spaciousness: ✵ ✵ ✵
Quiet: ✵ ✵ ✵ ✵
Security: ✵ ✵ ✵ ✵ ✵
Cleanliness: ✵ ✵ ✵ ✵ ✵

KEY INFORMATION

ADDRESS: 14548 Beaver Dam Ln., Plainview, IL

OPERATED BY: IDNR

CONTACT: (217) 854-8020, www.dnr.state.il .us/lands/land mgt/parks/r4/ beaver.htm

OPEN: Year-round

SITES: 18 Class B (tent) sites, 66 Class A (RV) sites, 1 cabin

EACH SITE: Electric (Class A only); picnic table, grill, and fire block; lantern pole (Class B only)

ASSIGNMENT: First come, first served; cabins reservable

REGISTRATION: With campground host, or at park office (if no host)

FACILITIES: Water spigots, vault toilets, shower house with flush toilets

PARKING: At campsite

FEE: Class B: $10 per night; Class A: $20 per night, $30 per night holidays; cabin: $40 per night plus $5 reservation fee

ELEVATION: 608 feet

RESTRICTIONS: *Pets:* On leash only
Fires: In fire rings only
Alcohol: Not allowed
Vehicles: 2 per site
Other: 14-day limit; 2 tents or 1 RV per site; 4 adults or 1 family per site

---

trails around it. You can host the gang for supper at your tent site, equipped with two tables and plenty of space. Or you can all eat on the patio overlooking the lake at the restaurant, open 6 a.m. to 7 p.m.

As you come up the hill from the lake, the road forks, entering the campground loop. Go left and you'll enter on the RV side. During camping season, you'll find the campground host by site 1, where you can register. Most of these sites are adequate for RVs, but lousy for tents. All have gravel pads and electrical hookups, with water spigots nearby, but are small and close together. Continue and you'll come to a small loop. If you must tent camp in this section, the sites on either side of the loop (15, 16, 17, 18, 24, 25, 26) are decent choices, with a bit more space and tree cover. You'll find a few more spacious RV sites if you head back to the T-intersection and turn left; these are 43, 44, and 47 on the outside of the loop.

Take the right fork from the lake (or follow the loop around from the RV side), and you'll enter the tent-camping section, with 18 sites. Most of these are refreshingly more spacious and spread out than the RV sites, though still open. All have two picnic tables, a fire block and grill, a lantern pole, and space for two vehicles. Sites 1, 2, and 3 are on a short spur, featuring some shade and a great view of the lake below. Together with sites 4 through 6 these are labeled "youth group area"; however, youth groups must reserve in advance, and if not reserved these are open for regular camping—check with the office. Sites 7 and 8 are the most spacious and separate, and either would be my first choice. If you need two adjacent sites, some seem to be naturally paired: 9 and 10, 12 and 14, 11 and 13, and 16 and 17. All are spacious—just closer to one another. Only sites 15 and 18 are too small.

The tent and RV sites are on the same loop, but on separate ridges, with a small wooded valley between them. You'll feel like it's a different camping area, but you're still just a short walk from the modern shower house, which tent campers can use.

Security is good here. The park is relatively small, with only a single entrance, so access is more controlled. A campground host is available round the clock

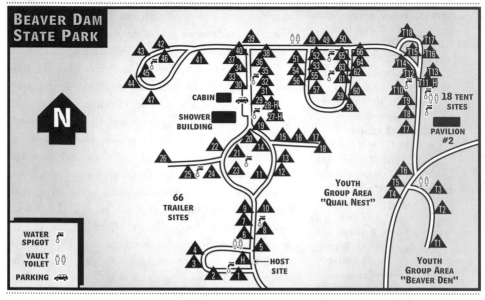

BEAVER DAM STATE PARK

in summer, and local law enforcement drive through at night. Even on weekends it's surprisingly quiet for such a popular place.

Beaver Dam opened in the 1890s as a private fishing club for local Carlinville businessmen, and fishing is still popular here today. You can purchase bait and tackle, as well as ice and some food and picnic supplies at the concession, open April to October. The lake is stocked with largemouth bass, bluegill, sunfish, and channel catfish. Trout are restocked the second Saturday in October—expect the lake to be busy that weekend.

GETTING THERE

From I-55 at IL 108 (Exit 60), take IL 108 west 11 miles to Carlinville. Go through Carlinville to the Amtrak station at Alton Road. Turn left and drive 7 miles to the Beaver Dam entrance on the right.

GPS COORDINATES

UTM Zone 16S
Easting 0243361
Northing 4343966
Latitude N 39° 12' 25.4751"
Longitude W 89° 58' 19.8892"

23
RAMSEY LAKE STATE PARK

> *Ramsey Lake is a fisherman's park, and multiple campgrounds offer some nice, quiet choices for tent campers.*

RAMSEY LAKE STATE PARK FEATURES 1,980 acres of wooded hills and valleys, with its beautiful 46-acre namesake lake as the centerpiece. Most people come here for the lake—fishing and boating are popular, and camping is almost as popular. There are multiple campgrounds, though, and most campers gravitate to the one best suited for RVs, leaving some nice quiet choices for tent campers.

First, the best choice. From the park entrance, take the first right and go north to the fork and left at the Pine Bend Campground sign. Because it is small—just six walk-in sites—this secluded area can occasionally fill up on weekends. But if it's not completely full, the sites are spacious enough so you'll have plenty of privacy—and midweek you could easily have it all to yourself. The two sites south of the loop are just 25 feet from parking and spread beneath two massive oaks. If you want to get farther from any casual traffic that might drive through to explore, settle at one of the four sites on the north side. The farthest is a 225-foot walk and has the best tree cover. All have a ground grill and table. Vault toilets are by the road, but you'll need to get water at one of the other campgrounds.

The second-best choice for tent camping is Hickory Grove Campground, with approximately 38 drive-in sites (my count—the park Web site says 45). From the park entrance, take the first right, then make a left and go past the group campground. Sites 112 through 130 are in the grass along the roadside, and you can park on the grass. Those on the right (112 through 120) have more shade and space, and 118, 119, and 120 are well away from the road. I like site 112, which is the farthest back and has mature tree cover. On the left, 121, 122, and 123 are sufficiently shaded and roomy; 127 through 130 are, by comparison, cramped. Farther down the road, sites 93 through 111 have gravel pull-ins. I don't

RATINGS

Beauty: ✩ ✩ ✩ ✩
Privacy: ✩ ✩ ✩
Spaciousness: ✩ ✩ ✩ ✩
Quiet: ✩ ✩ ✩ ✩
Security: ✩ ✩ ✩ ✩ ✩
Cleanliness: ✩ ✩ ✩ ✩ ✩

like these as well, except for 110, at the end of the loop to the right—it's large, and right by vault toilets and a small playground. All the sites have a ground grill and table, and most have a lantern pole. Hickory Grove is rarely more than half full, so you should be able to find a suitable site most weekends.

A third possibility is the group campground you pass on the way to Hickory Grove. These 24 sites are set up in groups of three and have tables, ground grills, and electricity, plus a big fire ring for each group. They're open to individual campers if not already taken or reserved by a group. Sites 22 through 24 are the best choice here—farthest from the road, with lots of room to spread out under the trees. They are reservable for $5 more per site; you must reserve a minimum of six sites.

White Oak is the Class A campground, with 90 electric sites, a rental cabin with bunk beds and electricity, and a shower house. From the park entrance, go straight to White Oak Campground on the right. This would be my last choice for tent camping, but it's the only option from December 1 to March 1, when the other campgrounds are closed. Whichever site you settle on, be sure to register at the park office (8 a.m. to 4 p.m.) or after hours with the campground host in White Oak (site 41, by the showers) before setting up. White Oak sites 1–30 and the cabin are reservable by mail and phone.

Ramsey Lake is a fisherman's park, and the lake is stocked with largemouth bass, bluegill, redear, channel catfish, and black crappie. There are five floating docks—off White Oak, Hickory Grove, and the youth group campgrounds—from which you can fish. The concession at the lake is under new management as of 2007, and they have greatly expanded their business. You can purchase ice, firewood, all sorts of fishing and camping supplies, basic groceries, snacks, and ice cream, as well as rent rowboats or paddleboats. Rowboats are $10 for eight hours without a motor, or $25 with a trolling motor; paddleboats are $5 per hour. Boat rental is brisk on weekends, so it's wise to call (618) 322-9766 to reserve one. They're usually open daily April through October from 7 a.m. to 5 p.m.

KEY INFORMATION

ADDRESS: Ramsey Lake Road, P.O. Box 97, Ramsey, IL 62080

OPERATED BY: IDNR

CONTACT: (618) 423-2215, www.dnr.state.il.us/lands/land mgt/parks/r5/ramsey.htm

OPEN: Year-round (White Oak only); other campgrounds closed at least Dec. 1–Mar. 1

SITES: Class D: 6 walk-in sites (Pine Bend); Class C: 38 sites (Hickory Grove); Class B: 24 group sites; Class A: 90 sites (White Oak); 1 cabin

EACH SITE: Picnic table, grill

ASSIGNMENT: First come, first served

REGISTRATION: At office or with campground host

FACILITIES: Water spigots, vault toilets, shower house (closed Dec. 1–Apr. 1)

PARKING: At site (Class A); in lot (Class D)

FEE: White Oak: $20/night, $30/night holidays; group: $18/night; Hickory Grove: $8/night; Pine Bend: $6/night; cabin: $45/night

ELEVATION: 619 feet

RESTRICTIONS: *Pets:* On leash only *Fires:* In fire rings *Alcohol:* Permitted *Vehicles:* 2 per site *Other:* 14 day limit; 1 RV or tent or 2 smaller tents per site; 4 adults or 1 family of 6 per site

MAP

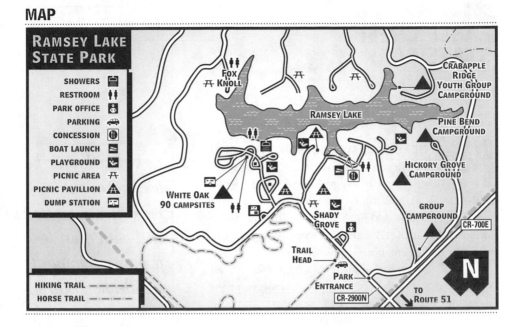

RAMSEY LAKE STATE PARK

SHOWERS	🚿
RESTROOM	🚻
PARK OFFICE	🏢
PARKING	🚗
CONCESSION	🏪
BOAT LAUNCH	🛥
PLAYGROUND	🛝
PICNIC AREA	🌲
PICNIC PAVILLION	⛺
DUMP STATION	🚐

FOX KNOLL

RAMSEY LAKE

CRABAPPLE RIDGE YOUTH GROUP CAMPGROUND

PINE BEND CAMPGROUND

HICKORY GROVE CAMPGROUND

WHITE OAK 90 CAMPSITES

SHADY GROVE

GROUP CAMPGROUND

CR-700E

TRAIL HEAD

PARK ENTRANCE

CR-2900N

TO ROUTE 51

N

HIKING TRAIL – – – – –
HORSE TRAIL – · – · –

GETTING THERE

On IL 51, go 15 miles south of Pana, or 13 miles north of the intersection of IL 51 and I-70 in Vandalia. Turn west onto CR 2900 at the brown park sign, then go 1 mile to the park entrance.

GPS COORDINATES

UTM Zone 16S
Easting 0316670
Northing 4336615
Latitude N 39° 9' 34.0163"
Longitude W 89° 7' 18.6536"

For hikers, there's a 1.8-mile loop trail, with trail-head parking by the office. Equestrians will find a small horse campground 1 mile north of the main park entrance, linked to a 15-mile loop that explores the terrain away from the lake.

Do take time for a slow drive on the scenic and hilly 4-mile loop around the lake (one-way clockwise). At the less visited rear section of the park, perched on ridges overlooking the lake, you'll find some nice picnic areas where you might be tempted to spend a few solitary hours enjoying the view, reading a book, or taking a nap.

I N 1963 THE U.S. ARMY CORPS OF ENGINEERS began work in central Illinois on a dam across the Kaskaskia River, with the goal of developing a new mid-state watershed and recreational lake. The result was long, narrow Lake Shelbyville, Illinois' third-largest lake, with 172 miles of shoreline offering a wide array of recreational opportunities.

That project has resulted in a huge lakeside leisure mecca, with hotels, restaurants, entertainment, shopping, marinas, fishing, and, of course, camping. There are at least 2,000 campsites in the public and private campgrounds scattered around the lake. And, as you might expect, most cater to the RV crowd.

Despite all this development, the area still hasn't lost its farming community, small-town charm. It's certainly not a Branson, or even a Lake of the Ozarks. Most visitors still come primarily for fishing, camping, swimming, or boating—in that order, according to a recent survey. The outdoors is still the main attraction and remains relatively unsullied by tourism.

If you'd like to enjoy Lake Shelbyville while tent camping, there are some good options. Two state parks sit across the lake from each other—Wolf Creek State Park (on the eastern shore) and Eagle Creek State Park (on the western)— and both have tent-camping areas. Choosing between the two is difficult, but Eagle Creek gets my vote, at least for camping. Eagle Creek's campground is smaller by half—smaller means fewer people. Also, Eagle Creek isn't generally as busy, its tent area is separate from the RV section, and the sites themselves are farther from one another.

As you enter the campground, pass the check-in station and turn left. Proceed 0.5 miles. Make the next right, and you'll enter the parking lot for the walk-in tent sites; go straight, and you'll enter the spur for the drive-in tent sites.

> *Lake Shelbyville has become an outdoor recreational mecca but still hasn't lost its farming community, small-town charm.*

RATINGS

Beauty: ✿ ✿ ✿ ✿
Privacy: ✿ ✿ ✿
Spaciousness: ✿ ✿ ✿
Quiet: ✿ ✿ ✿ ✿
Security: ✿ ✿ ✿ ✿
Cleanliness: ✿ ✿ ✿

KEY INFORMATION

ADDRESS: RR 1 Box 198B, Findlay, IL 62534

OPERATED BY: IDNR

CONTACT: (217) 756-8260, www.dnr.state.il.us/lands/land mgt/parks/r3/eaglecrk.htm

OPEN: Year-round

SITES: Class C: 11 walk-in tent sites, 15 drive-in tent sites; Class A: 148 sites

EACH SITE: Picnic table, fire ring; electric (Class A only)

ASSIGNMENT: First come, first served; Class A sites 1–56 and walk-in sites T2–T6 reservable by mail

REGISTRATION: Set up and park staff will come by or register with campground host

FACILITIES: Water spigots, vault toilets, shower house

PARKING: At site; at lot

FEE: Class A: $20 per night, $30 on holidays; Class C drive-in: $10 per night; Class C walk-in: $8 per night; $5 reservation fee

ELEVATION: 663 feet

RESTRICTIONS: *Pets:* On leash only *Fires:* In fire rings only *Alcohol:* Permitted *Vehicles:* 2 per site *Other:* 14-day limit; 2 tents or 1 RV per site; 4 adults or 1 family per site

Each tent section stretches along a separate, wooded ridge with plenty of shade and ends on a beautiful point overlooking the lake. In many campgrounds that have both walk-in and drive-in tent sites, the walk-ins tend to be more spacious and scenic—you get some perks for carrying your gear from the parking area. At Eagle Creek, however, I like the drive-in sites better. Of the 15 drive-in sites, 10, 12, 13, and 14 are a bit too small and close together. Site 2 is the most spacious, and site 15 is the most scenic and separate, being at the end of the point.

The walk-in tent section is similarly arranged, with 11 sites. These are a bit closer together and more open than the drive-in sites. The closest is just 30 feet from the parking lot, while the farthest is about 300 feet away. Again, the nicest is at the end of the point, site T11.

The tent sites are equipped with a table, a fire ring with grill, and a lamp pole; vault toilets and water spigots are by the entrance. Tent campers can also use the modern shower house in the RV section. You can reserve sites T2 throughT6 in the walk-in area by mail, but it simply isn't necessary. The tent areas never fill up, and an average busy weekend sees only about five sites occupied.

If you turn right at the campground check-in, you'll enter the 148-site RV section, where there are electrical hookups. If you'd prefer to camp in this area, go straight back to the dead-end loop around sites 146 through 148, where you'll find more space and less traffic.

While at Eagle Creek, don't miss the chance to hike along the lakeshore and admire the views. You can choose between 0.5-mile High Bluff Trail, a loop beginning near site 96 in the RV campground, and 11-mile Chief Illini Trail, which begins across the park road from the tent-camping area.

Whether you own or rent a boat, or prefer to stick to the banks, fishing is huge at Lake Shelbyville, which is home to crappie, largemouth bass, walleye, channel and flathead catfish, bluegill, muskie, bullhead, carp, and sunfish. And for just $1, you can swim all day at one of the four public beaches around the lake. The closest is at Wolf Creek State Park, 9 miles away. Beaches and pools are usually open Memorial Day to

MAP

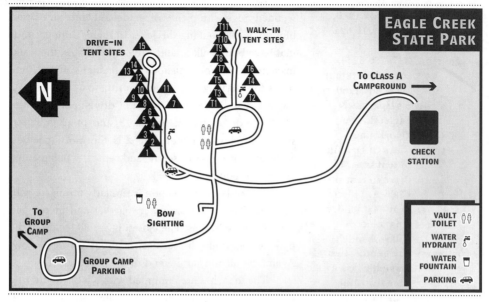

Labor Day, but in recent years low water levels have delayed beach openings, so call or check online first.

If you want a break from the rustic, head south in the park to Eagle Creek Resort. Here you can relax before the lobby fireplace and eat at Bunker's Bar & Grille (open during the summer) or at the fancier Rosewood. There are indoor and outdoor pools, which campers can use for $5 per day, plus a very popular 18-hole golf course—you should call well in advance to reserve a tee-time. (The mini-golf, bike, and boat rentals here are only for resort guests.)

See **www.lakeshelbyville.com** and **www.mvs.usace .army.mil/shelbyville** for more information on area attractions.

GETTING THERE

From Decatur, take IL 121 south to IL 128 in Dalton City. Turn right, go 14 miles south to Findlay Road (CR 2100 North), and turn left. Drive 4 miles to the Eagle Creek sign (CR 2200 East), and turn right. Head 0.75 miles, turn left at the sign, and go 1 mile to the park entrance.

GPS COORDINATES

UTM Zone 16S
Easting 0352205
Northing 4374777
Latitude N 39° 30' 35.7184"
Longitude W 88° 43' 8.9767"

> *The campgrounds at Walnut Point provide easy access for fishing or boating and afford a scenic view right from your campsite.*

LIKE THE FINGERS OF AN OUTSTRETCHED HAND, the little peninsulas on which the campgrounds at Walnut Point State Park are situated jut out into the beautiful 60-acre lake, providing easy access for fishing or boating, and affording a scenic view right from your campsite. In some cases you can row up to your site or fish at a dock just a few steps from your tent. This small park boasts 60 sites, but they are spread out in separate loops, so they don't have the typical "sardines-in-a-can" campground feel. The tent-only campsites are walk-ins—close enough to parking to be convenient but far enough that they're not as popular as the pull-in sites. And tent campers can use the showers—a nice perk.

Enter Walnut Point from the north, turn left, and follow the loop around the lake to the back of the park, where the campgrounds are. Over the dam and past the concession, you'll see the entrance to Fox Squirrel Campground. Pull-in sites 1 through 14 are on this drive; parking for the walk-in tent sites is just opposite site 10, along with a water spigot and vault toilets.

Past Fox Squirrel is the modern shower house, which all campers can use. Farther on the right you'll see parking for the Gray Tent walk-in sites, and beyond that, at the end of the road, you'll find the Gray Squirrel pull-in sites.

The best choices for tent camping are the 20 walk-in sites in the Fox Tent and Gray Tent areas. All have two picnic tables, a wood-chipped tent pad, a ground grill or fire ring, and a lantern post. Holidays may find these areas fairly full, but less than half will be occupied on most other good camping weekends.

Walk 250 feet from the Fox Tent parking lot to the end of the peninsula, where you'll see lots of space surrounding sites 7 and 8, the two most scenic sites in this area. Here you'll find plenty of shade, an

RATINGS

Beauty: ✩ ✩ ✩ ✩
Privacy: ✩ ✩ ✩ ✩
Spaciousness: ✩ ✩ ✩ ✩
Quiet: ✩ ✩ ✩ ✩
Security: ✩ ✩ ✩ ✩
Cleanliness: ✩ ✩ ✩ ✩

unobstructed view of the lake, and a dock right off site 7. Site 5 is a bit farther back from the trail than the others. Site 1 is wheelchair accessible, and just behind site 2 is an accessible dock and fishing platform.

I like the sites in Gray Tent best. Site 20, a 350-foot walk to the end of the peninsula, boasts a great view and plenty of room to spread out. If you want something a bit closer, sites 11 and 13 are less than 100 feet from parking, off a dogleg to the right of the trail. These feel more secluded. Site 13 also has a dock and is the single most popular of all the walk-ins; it was occupied 65 nights in 2007. If your group needs two adjacent sites, check out the combination of sites 16 and 18, which are close to one another but separate from the others.

If you want electricity, the best Class A sites are at the back of the Gray Squirrel loop—sites 15, 17, and 19 on the outside of the loop offer ample space for a tent, shade, and proximity to the lake; there's a dock just behind site 15. The sites in Fox Squirrel loop are not as spacious; site 5 is probably the best choice there for space and shade, though it's close to the restroom.

If you want a pull-in site but don't need electricity, sites B1 through B6 at the entrance to the Gray Squirrel loop aren't bad. B1, B2, and B3 have space for a pop-up trailer to back in and feature a cleared, wood-chipped pad for a tent.

Walnut Point is one of the rare Illinois state parks where most sites are reservable—and where it might pay to reserve on a prime camping weekend. Check the park Web site for the necessary form, which you have to print and mail in with the $5 reservation fee. (Only the Class B sites can't be reserved.)

If you like woodland hikes with a destination, the longest trail at Walnut Point features a unique sight. Take the aptly named Whispering Pines Trail counterclockwise, and watch for the signs for Observatory Trail. This 2.55-mile loop leads you past a three-story domed concrete bunker: an observatory built by the University of Illinois in the late 1960s. While it no longer functions and you can't go in, it is interesting and unusual to see.

The concession at Shady Bay serves as a popular gathering point and is open from mid-April to the end of

KEY INFORMATION

ADDRESS: 2331 East County Road 370 North, Oakland, IL 61943

OPERATED BY: IDNR

CONTACT: (217) 346-3336, www.dnr.state.il.us/lands/landmgt/parks/r3/walnutpt.htm

OPEN: Year-round

SITES: Class C: 20 walk-in sites; Class B: 6 sites; Class A: 34 electric sites

EACH SITE: Picnic tables, fire ring and grate

ASSIGNMENT: First come, first served; reservations available by mail for Class A and C

REGISTRATION: Register with campground host or set up and park staff will come by

FACILITIES: Water spigots, vault toilets, shower house

PARKING: At site (Class A & B); at lot (Class C)

FEE: Class A: $20 per night, $30 per night on holidays; Class B: $13 per night; Class C: $8 per night; $5 reservation fee

ELEVATION: 657 feet

RESTRICTIONS: *Pets:* On leash only
Fires: In fire rings only
Alcohol: Not permitted at Class C sites
Vehicles: 2 per site
Other: 14-day limit; 1 RV and 1 tent, or 2 tents per site; 4 adults or 1 family per site; no swimming

MAP

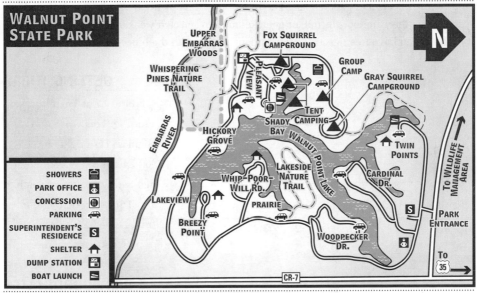

WALNUT POINT STATE PARK

N

UPPER EMBARRAS WOODS

WHISPERING PINES NATURE TRAIL

FOX SQUIRREL CAMPGROUND

GROUP CAMP

GRAY SQUIRREL CAMPGROUND

PLEASANT VIEW

TENT CAMPING

SHADY BAY

HICKORY GROVE

EMBARRAS RIVER

WALNUT POINT LAKE

TWIN POINTS

CARDINAL DR.

TO WILDLIFE MANAGEMENT AREA

LAKESIDE NATURE TRAIL

WHIP-POOR-WILL RD.

LAKEVIEW

PRAIRIE

BREEZY POINT

WOODPECKER DR.

PARK ENTRANCE

TO 35

CR-7

SHOWERS	
PARK OFFICE	
CONCESSION	
PARKING	
SUPERINTENDENT'S RESIDENCE	S
SHELTER	
DUMP STATION	
BOAT LAUNCH	

MAP

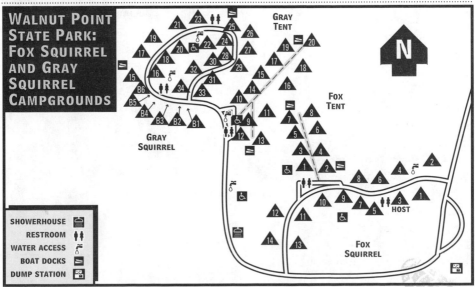

WALNUT POINT STATE PARK: FOX SQUIRREL AND GRAY SQUIRREL CAMPGROUNDS

N

GRAY TENT

FOX TENT

GRAY SQUIRREL

HOST

FOX SQUIRREL

SHOWERHOUSE	
RESTROOM	
WATER ACCESS	
BOAT DOCKS	
DUMP STATION	

October every day from 8 a.m. to 9 p.m. There you can purchase firewood, ice, and bait, and rent rowboats and paddleboats. The restaurant offers plenty of snack and meal choices; you can eat there, indoors or out, or get take-out. On selected weekends from May to October they even have free musical entertainment—check with the office for a schedule.

GETTING THERE

From I-57 at Tuscola, take Exit 212. Follow US 36 East 13 miles. Turn right onto CR 2360 East at the Walnut Point sign and drive 6 miles south. Turn right onto CR 400 North. Drive 0.25 miles to the park entrance, on the left.

GPS COORDINATES

UTM Zone 16S
Easting 0411658
Northing 4395534
Latitude N 39° 42' 18.3280"
Longitude W 88° 1' 49.8161"

Marshall

> *Hike among the smooth gray beech trees, little changed since the days when the Lincolns passed this way.*

RATINGS

Beauty: ✪ ✪ ✪ ✪
Privacy: ✪ ✪
Spaciousness: ✪ ✪ ✪
Quiet: ✪ ✪ ✪ ✪
Security: ✪ ✪ ✪ ✪ ✪
Cleanliness: ✪ ✪ ✪ ✪ ✪

ILLINOIS IS KNOWN AS THE "LAND OF LINCOLN," and many sites around the state commemorate events from the life of the state's most famous resident to reach the White House. Fifty years after Lincoln's death, the state decided to mark the exact route traveled by Lincoln's family when they moved from Kentucky to Illinois. Eventually the 1,000-mile Lincoln Trail was established, and the state park of the same name lies just west of the trail as it follows Illinois Route 1.

Lincoln Trail State Park covers more than 1,000 acres of densely wooded hills and ravines around a U-shaped 146-acre lake. It's a beautiful destination for hiking, boating, and fishing, and offers two very different campgrounds with some scenic tent-camping spots. Add some luxuries like an excellent shower house and a great restaurant, and it's worth spending a relaxing weekend here.

As you enter, stop first at the park office to register for a campsite, unless the sign posted says otherwise. Then turn left on the loop road that encircles the lake to head toward the campgrounds. The first entrance on the left is for the impeccable but aptly named Plainview Campground. Plainview has 129 sites neatly arranged in open grassy sections. Everything is well manicured and clean, including the almost new shower building (redone in 2004). But your view will be of the rows of surrounding RVs, and the young trees have not yet come into their own for shade. Most sites are electric, except for sites 38 through 50 (even) and 87 through 93 (odd) on the east side. If you want an electric site here, try for one of the pull-through sites—2 through 12 (even)—which offer the most shade and space.

Lincoln Trail's second campground, Lakeside, is just down the road on the right, and it's starkly different. Here you'll find plenty of mature woods and, appropriately enough, some great views of the lake that surrounds it on three sides. Most of the 99 sites have electrical hookups and pull-in gravel pads, but 26 walk-in tent-only sites are scattered among them in small pockets. The tent sites are 30 through 33, 61 through 65, 66 through 72, 73, 74, 84 through 87, and 92 through 95. Each is a short walk from the adjacent parking area and has a table, ground grill, and lantern pole. All are on the lake, but my favorites are 84 through 87, which have nice flat tent pads, and 61 through 65, which have towering trees for shade. If you need two sites, grab 73 and 74, and you'll have the spot all to yourselves. If you want electricity, I recommend site 13, which is beautiful, overlooking a ravine, and is right by the entrance to Beech Tree Trail, or else sites 45, 46, or 88 through 91, which are right on the lake. There are water spigots and vault toilets throughout, and all campers can use the showers in Plainview (closed mid-November to late March). The sites in the tent areas are a bit close together and might feel crowded on a really busy weekend, but this campground almost never fills up, least of all the walk-in sites.

Behind site 14 in Lakeside Campground, you can pick up the scenic 0.5-mile Beech Tree Trail, which proceeds along wooden stairways and bridges and down to the lake. Along the way you'll skirt the American Beech Woods nature preserve, passing among the smooth, gray beech trees that have changed little from the days when the Lincolns passed this way. The reward at the end is Lincoln Trail's excellent and popular restaurant, which features dinners, sandwiches, a salad bar, ice cream, and specials, and is open 365 days a year, from 6 a.m. to 8 p.m. Even if you do all your own campfire cooking, the view of the lake from the restaurant makes it worth coming in just for pie and coffee. The marina and bait shop downstairs are open May to October (depending on the weather); you can purchase fishing supplies, snacks, ice, and firewood, and rent rowboats, pontoon boats, and paddleboats here. Fishing is good, and the 7 miles of wooded shoreline are well worth exploring. You'll need to bring your own motor, though, 10 horsepower or under.

KEY INFORMATION

ADDRESS:	16985 East 1350th Rd., Marshall, IL
OPERATED BY:	IDNR
CONTACT:	(217) 826-2222, www.dnr.state.il.us/lands/land mgt/parks/r3/lincoln.htm
OPEN:	Year-round
SITES:	Class C: 27 walk-in tent sites; Class B: 11 non-electric sites; Class A: 190 electric sites
EACH SITE:	Picnic table, fire ring and grate; electric at Class A only
ASSIGNMENT:	First come, first served
REGISTRATION:	Register at office unless posted
FACILITIES:	Water spigots, vault toilets, shower house (closed Nov.–Mar.)
PARKING:	At site (Class A & B); in lot (Class C)
FEE:	Class A: $20 per night, $30 per night holidays; Class B: $10 per night; Class C: $8 per night; $2 less when showers are closed
ELEVATION:	633 feet
RESTRICTIONS:	*Pets:* On leash only *Fires:* In fire rings only *Alcohol:* Permitted *Vehicles:* 2 per site *Other:* 14-day limit; 1 RV and 1 tent, or 2 tents per site; 4 adults or 1 family per site

MAP

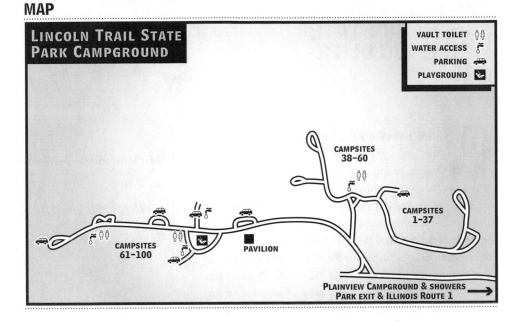

LINCOLN TRAIL STATE PARK CAMPGROUND

VAULT TOILET
WATER ACCESS
PARKING
PLAYGROUND

CAMPSITES 38-60

CAMPSITES 1-37

CAMPSITES 61-100

PAVILION

PLAINVIEW CAMPGROUND & SHOWERS
PARK EXIT & ILLINOIS ROUTE 1 →

GETTING THERE

From I-70, take Exit 147 at Marshall to IL 1. Go 5.2 miles south to CR 1350 North. Turn right and drive 1 mile to the park entrance.

GPS COORDINATES

UTM Zone 16S
Easting 0439384
Northing 4355493
Latitude N 39° 20' 48.3099"
Longitude W 87° 42' 12.4585"

If you want more hiking, try the 2-mile Sand Ford Nature Trail in the southwest corner of the park. You can get even more of a workout on the 8-mile trail system at Fox Ridge State Park, about 30 miles to the west. The camping there is best left to RVs, but the hiking is rigorous, scenic, and well worth the side trip. Fox Ridge consists of a series of ravines along a glacial moraine, so the trails include lots of ups and downs, with many wooden stairs and bridges to help. If you go there, be sure to scale the 144 steps to the Eagle's Nest deck, overlooking the Embarras (pronounced "ambraw") River. Fox Ridge is about 6 miles south of Charleston on IL 130.

SAM PARR STATE FISH & WILDLIFE AREA

WHEN I WAS A KID, I never understood how my great-grandfather could sit fishing for hours, even with nothing biting. I realize now that fishing was just an excuse for enjoying the outdoors, and whether the fish cooperated or not was immaterial. I'm reminded of that because Sam Parr State Fish & Wildlife Area is just a few miles from where my great-grandfather lived most of his life and is just the sort of peaceful place he loved. The terrain is typical of central Illinois—a mix of low timbered hills and prairie, with a narrow V-shaped 183-acre lake at the center. The park doesn't have a lot of amenities, but the separate tent-camping area offers quiet lakeside camping and a good place to enjoy fishing, boating, and simply relaxing.

As you enter Sam Parr off IL 33, go 0.3 miles, to the second road on the right, and follow the signs for tent camping. The walk-in tent area is at the southwest corner of the lake and has 21 sites spread out over a large grassy lawn sloping gently toward the lake. Though all the sites are visible to one another, most are spacious and widely separated. Some are close to parking, so you don't have to carry your gear very far at all, while those on the lakeshore require a short hike of 300 to 450 feet. Most of the time you should have plenty of choices. The walk-in area is busy on holidays, but other weekends may only see two or three parties camping, and it's rarely even half full.

Site 1 is attractive but too close to the parking lot for my comfort—you'll see and hear everyone who drives in. If you want to be close to your vehicle, try sites 2, 3, 11, or 14, which are a bit farther and shaded by pine or maple trees. I prefer the sites on the fringes (out of the line of foot traffic) and closest to the lake. Sites 6, 8, 9, 10, 16, and 20 all fit the bill. Site 8 is on a bit of a slope but is pretty and well shaded. My favorites are site 9—not

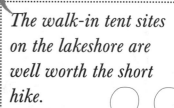

The walk-in tent sites on the lakeshore are well worth the short hike.

RATINGS

Beauty: ✩ ✩ ✩ ✩
Privacy: ✩ ✩ ✩
Spaciousness: ✩ ✩ ✩ ✩
Quiet: ✩ ✩ ✩ ✩
Security: ✩ ✩ ✩ ✩
Cleanliness: ✩ ✩ ✩ ✩ ✩

ADDRESS: 13225 East State Highway 33, Newton, IL 62448

OPERATED BY: IDNR

CONTACT: (618) 783-2661, www.dnr.state.il .us/lands/land mgt/parks/r5/ samparr.htm

OPEN: Year-round

SITES: Class D: 21 walk-in tent sites; Class B/E: 33 electric sites

EACH SITE: Picnic table, fire ring or ground grill; electric in Class B/E only

ASSIGNMENT: First come, first served

REGISTRATION: Register at the office after selecting site

FACILITIES: Water spigots, vault toilets

PARKING: At site (Class B/E); in lot (Class D)

FEE: Class B/E: $18 per night; Class D: $6 per night

ELEVATION: 523 feet

RESTRICTIONS: *Pets:* On leash only *Fires:* In fire rings only *Alcohol:* Permitted *Vehicles:* 2 per site *Other:* 14-day limit; 1 RV and 1 tent, or 2 tents per site; 4 adults or 1 family per site

much shade but a beautiful view of the lake, and right by a little fishing dock—and site 20. They're the farthest from parking but well worth the extra steps.

Each site has a table and a fire ring or a ground grill; vault toilets and a water spigot are located near the parking lot. Only the water spigot at the park office is open in winter. Once you've selected a site, register at the office, on the first road to the right as you enter the park.

The RV campground, with 33 electric sites, is at the end of the park road, to the north and around the lake. The location is beautiful—a wooded peninsula between the arms of the lake—but the sites are small, with gravel pads and not a lot of tent space.

Sam Parr has 2 miles of foot trails, and the nicest section, along the lakeshore, begins at the dam on the southern end. There are two boat ramps, but no boat rental or concession.

If you enjoy natural history, check out Prairie Ridge State Natural Area, about 10 miles southwest of Sam Parr. These 4,100 acres of tall prairie and marsh are the last Illinois refuge of the once-abundant prairie chicken and home to numerous other state endangered or threatened species. From late March through April, you may be privileged to witness the loud "booming" of the male prairie chicken's courtship dance. Limited access means roadside viewing, except around the office and in the portion owned by the Illinois Audubon Society. To get to the Prairie Ridge office from Sam Parr, take IL 33 2.5 miles into Newton, then turn left onto Liberty Street (1100 East). Drive 3.8 miles south to 600 North, turn right, go 1 mile west to 1000 East, turn left, and travel 1.75 miles south to the white house with the wire fence. The Audubon Society parking area, with trails and an observation deck, is 0.25 miles farther south, then 0.6 miles east. For more information, see **www.dnr.state.il.us/ORC/prairieridge/index.htm.**

For more-conventional history, visit the Lincoln Log Cabin State Historic Site, 30 miles north of Sam Parr. The site includes a replica of the log cabin in which Abe Lincoln's father and stepmother lived when they moved to Illinois in 1837, as well as a working period farm. Costumed site interpreters present pioneer life,

MAP

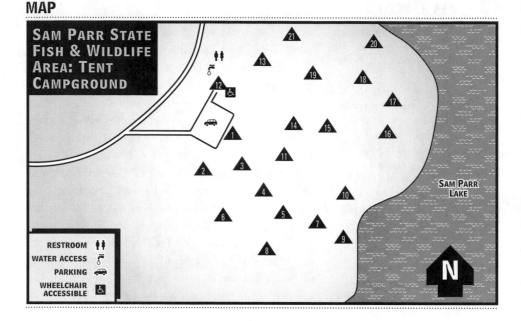

and, on a given day, you may witness shearing sheep, carding wool, harvesting wheat, or making brooms, or may even witness the visit of an itinerant 19th-century physician. The site is open Wednesday through Sunday from 8:30 a.m. to dusk. From Sam Parr, head 23.5 miles north on IL 130 to 1200 North—watch for a "Lincoln Cabin" sign. Turn left, go 4 miles west to 1450 East, then turn right and follow the road 2.6 miles north to the main entrance. Check **www.lincolnlogcabin.org** for more information.

GETTING THERE

From I-70 at Greenup, take Exit 119 and drive 17 miles south on IL 130 to IL 33. Turn left and go 0.75 miles to park entrance, on the left.

GPS COORDINATES

UTM Zone 16S
Easting 0402453
Northing 4318768
Latitude N 39° 0' 45.0199"
Longitude W 88° 7' 36.1081"

" *Don't miss the excellent sandy beach at Rocky Point.* "

THE STEPHEN A. FORBES State Recreation Area offers tent camping with some luxury and plenty of convenient recreation for families. The separate walk-in tent area gets you away from the busy main campground, but nearby you still have showers, swimming, boating, a restaurant, and even a small store. It doesn't hurt that the park's 585-acre lake is beautiful, with 18 miles of timbered shoreline and more than 1,100 acres of surrounding forest to explore if you want more nature and fewer people.

Whether you enter Forbes from the east or west, turn left and follow the main road around the lake to the northwest and the Oak Ridge Campground. Chances are good that most if not all of the 115 sites here will be occupied by RVs on any weekend. Continue straight south through the campground, passing the shower house, playground, and pavilion, to reach the small parking lot for walk-in tent campers. There are only ten sites here, spaced along a couple of short trails that head into the woods. This part of the campground is quieter and not nearly as busy. You might have it all to yourself midweek, and on non-holiday weekends usually no more than half the sites will be occupied.

You can park next to the closest sites, and the farthest is an easy walk of about 500 feet. You couldn't really call them isolated—the woods aren't dense, and there's not a lot of undergrowth separating the individual sites. Still, they're well shaded and about 75 to 100 feet from each other, which is much better than in the main campground. I prefer the farthest one, site 10, which offers the most space and the least chance that anyone will camp nearby. Sites 5 through 9 are all acceptable. Sites 3 and 4 are closer to each other, and 1 and 2 are too close to the parking lot. When I was there, site 1 was also muddy, even though none of the others were. If you want to stick close to your car, try

RATINGS

Beauty: ✩ ✩ ✩ ✩
Privacy: ✩ ✩ ✩ ✩
Spaciousness: ✩ ✩ ✩
Quiet: ✩ ✩ ✩ ✩
Security: ✩ ✩ ✩ ✩ ✩
Cleanliness: ✩ ✩ ✩ ✩ ✩

site 6 instead. Once you've selected a site, register with the host at the campground entrance.

Continue down the trail about 500 feet past site 10 to reach the lake. Here you connect with the 2.5-mile Oak Ridge loop trail, which goes around the point and through the main campground. You can hike it either direction and, if you don't want to do the whole loop, return to your campsite via the campground road.

The lake is the star attraction at Forbes. There's an excellent 200-foot sandy beach at Rocky Point, on the southeastern corner, where you can swim all day for $1 per person. The beach is open every day from Memorial Day weekend to Labor Day, weather permitting, from 10 a.m. (9 a.m. on weekends) to sunset. At the opposite corner of the lake, across the inlet from the campground, the marina rents motorized johnboats, pedal boats, and waterbikes. This is one of the few Illinois state park lakes with no horsepower limit, and about 1 mile of its length is open to waterskiing.

Anglers go for bluegill, crappie, and channel catfish on the lake, but it's especially known for largemouth bass. You can bank fish from the docks at the campgrounds, or from any of the picnic areas around the southern end of the lake. There are fish-cleaning stations at the campground entrance and at the Lakeview boat ramp on the east side.

After working up an appetite swimming, boating, fishing, or hiking, cross the inlet via the floating walkway to The Leaky Bucket restaurant, by the marina. This is one of the most attractive concession buildings I've seen at any Illinois park, with its landscaped waterfront, large dining room, and big picture windows overlooking the lake. The menu includes a decent selection of sandwiches, salads, and dinners, and, in keeping with the restaurant's name, several "bucket of" items—a bucket of fried mushrooms, apple fritters, onion rings, or catfish curls. Breakfast is available on the weekends, along with evening specials: Friday is all-you-can-eat fish, Saturday is prime rib or ribeye, and Sunday lunch is all-you-can-eat fried chicken. The Leaky Bucket is open every day but Monday from April 1 through November 1 from 7 a.m. to 7 p.m. (9 p.m. on Friday and Saturday). The attached store carries fishing,

KEY INFORMATION

ADDRESS: 6924 Omega Rd., Kinmundy, IL

OPERATED BY: IDNR

CONTACT: (618) 547-3381, www.dnr.state.il.us/lands/landmgt/parks/r5/stephen.htm

OPEN: Year-round

SITES: Class C: 10 walk-in sites; Class B: 5 non-electric sites; Class A: 110 electric sites; 1 cabin

EACH SITE: Picnic table, ground grill

ASSIGNMENT: First come, first served; cabin reservable

REGISTRATION: Register with campground host

FACILITIES: Water spigots, vault toilets, shower house (closed mid-Jan.–Apr. 15)

PARKING: At site (Class A and B); in lot (Class C)

FEE: Class A: $20 per night, $30 per night holidays; Class B: $10 per night; Class C: $8 per night; cabin: $45 per night ($5 reservation fee)

ELEVATION: 559 feet

RESTRICTIONS: *Pets:* On leash only *Fires:* In fire rings only *Alcohol:* Permitted *Vehicles:* 2 per site *Other:* 14-day limit; 1 camping unit (RV or tent) or 2 smaller tents per site; 4 adults or 1 family of 6 per site

MAP

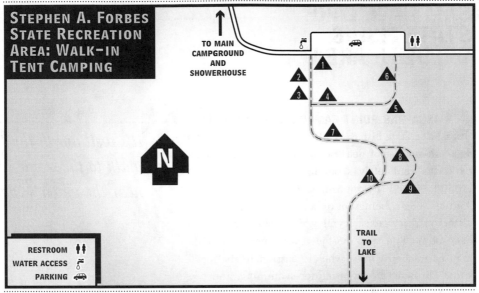

STEPHEN A. FORBES
STATE RECREATION
AREA: WALK-IN
TENT CAMPING

TO MAIN
CAMPGROUND
AND
SHOWERHOUSE

N

TRAIL
TO
LAKE

RESTROOM
WATER ACCESS
PARKING

GETTING THERE

From I-57, take Exit 127 and head east on Kinoka Road 1.25 miles to Broom Road (CR 1475). Turn right and go 1.55 miles south to Williams Road (CR 1800). Turn left and drive 4.25 miles east to Omega Road (CR 27). Turn right and the park entrance is 1 mile straight ahead.

GPS COORDINATES

UTM Zone 16S
Easting 0345230
Northing 4287881
Latitude N 38° 43' 33.7646"
Longitude W 88° 46' 49.5916"

camping, and boating supplies, as well as limited groceries and deli items. For more information, call (618) 547-9090.

If you're up for a challenging hike, about 20 miles north of Forbes is Wildcat Hollow, which seems like a piece of the Shawnee Forest transplanted north. The approximately 2.5-mile loop trail winds through upland forest, small canyons, and rocky streambeds—it starts easy, then gets rugged. You're sure to see wildlife—just don't go during deer-hunting season. Pick up a trail map at the Forbes office. To get there, head north to IL 37, turn right, then continue about 14 miles to Mason. Turn left on Main Street (CR 24), go 1.3 miles north, and turn right at the first intersection after I-57. Turn left on the gravel road and follow it to the parking lot.

SASSAFRAS POINT CAMPGROUND at Sam Dale Lake State Fish & Wildlife Area ranks very high on my list of near-perfect tent spots in a state park. It's completely separate from the RV campgrounds—it's on the opposite side of the lake, in fact. And it's scenic, being out on a point, meaning there's water on three sides. Its 21 walk-in sites are spread out, not in a line, with most just far enough from parking to attract only those who are passionate about privacy. Throw in a free beach for swimming, and you have an ideal place for a relaxed getaway.

As you enter the park, go about 1.25 miles, heading past several roads to the right and the park office to the left, and turn right at the sign for Sassafras Point. There's a single parking lot and 21 amply shaded walk-in sites. Some sites are close to one another, but this campground is barely half full on a typical non-holiday weekend, so you shouldn't have to camp too near anyone else. You can go ahead and set up, and park personnel will come by later.

Most of these are great sites. Only 4 and 5 are too small; 7, 8, and 9 are in a line, so you risk anyone camping farther down the point walking through your camp. If you don't want to carry your gear far, sites 1 and 20 are right by the road—pull to the side, unload, and then park. The only downside is being right next to everyone coming in and out. A bit farther out and well shaded are sites 3 and 21, both great choices. Sites 10, 13, and 17 are excellent, and 12, 14, and 15, closest to the water's edge, are near perfect. Site 12 is the farthest, well worth the 275-foot walk. It is close to 11, but if you get 12, you can hope that no other camping isolationist will take 11. On the water's edge is a bench, where at night I watched the sun go down over the lake, and in the morning sipped coffee while great blue herons swooped down from the trees to fish in the shallows.

> *It's well worth the walk to the scenic sites near the water's edge.*

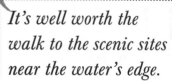

RATINGS

Beauty: ✩ ✩ ✩ ✩
Privacy: ✩ ✩ ✩ ✩
Spaciousness: ✩ ✩ ✩ ✩
Quiet: ✩ ✩ ✩ ✩
Security: ✩ ✩ ✩ ✩ ✩
Cleanliness: ✩ ✩ ✩ ✩ ✩

KEY INFORMATION

ADDRESS: R.R. 1, Johnsonville, IL 62850

OPERATED BY: IDNR

CONTACT: (618) 835-2292, www.dnr.state.il.us/lands/landmgt/parks/r5/samdale.htm

OPEN: Year-round

SITES: Class C: 21 walk-in sites; Class B/E: 66 electric sites; group campground

EACH SITE: Picnic table, ground grill; electric in Class B/E only

ASSIGNMENT: First come, first served; 12 sites reservable in Lakeview Campground

REGISTRATION: Set up first; park staff will come by or go to the campground host at Hickory Hollow

FACILITIES: Water spigots, vault toilets, swimming beach

PARKING: At site; in lot (walk-in sites)

FEE: Class B/E: $18 per night; Class C: $6 per night

ELEVATION: 489 feet

RESTRICTIONS: *Pets:* On leash only
Fires: In fire rings only
Alcohol: Permitted (except at beach)
Vehicles: 2 per site
Other: 14-day limit; 1 RV and 1 tent, or 2 tents per site; 4 adults or 1 family per site

If a perfect campsite isn't enough, just down the road from Sassafras Point and across the dam is an excellent beach, open from Memorial Day to Labor Day. The sign says it's open from sunrise to sunset, but, in fact, you can go anytime, even for a midnight swim—and it's free! Who needs showers when you can take a cool dip on a hot summer day?

Another nice option for privacy is the group campground, to the right as you enter the park. It's labeled "youth group" on the map but is available for any group, adults or just a family, from a handful to 50. It's not quite as attractive as Sassafras Point but is on the lake and has tables, grills, toilets, and water. You have to pay for a minimum of ten people ($4 per adult), no matter how small your group, but that might be well worth it if you want a place all to yourselves. It can be reserved, or you can register on arrival at the park office, if it's not already taken.

If you absolutely must have electricity, there are two Class B campgrounds past the beach. Hickory Hollow (labeled "A" on the park map) is the better choice, offering 32 wooded sites in a single loop. Of these, the sites at the outside back of the loop (11, 13, 14, and 15) seem less crunched together. Lakeview ("B" on the map) is the other campground. At the end of the road, it is the busiest, probably because 12 of its 34 sites are reservable.

On the road next to Sassafras Point you'll find the "Middle of Nowhere"—that's the name of the park's concession. Amazingly, they're open every day from mid-April through Columbus Day, 7 a.m. to 7:30 p.m., and you can pick up ice, firewood, bait, and limited camping and fishing supplies. You can rent a boat for an hour or overnight, but bring your own motor (under 10 horsepower). If you're tired of campfire cooking, the little restaurant offers a decent selection of sandwiches, salads, homemade pie, and nightly specials. As you're packing up to leave on a Sunday, take advantage of their fried-chicken buffet. And if you're an inveterate carnivore, you might just have to try the bison burger.

Anglers will enjoy fishing 194-acre Sam Dale Lake, whether by boat or along the shoreline from one of the picnic or camping areas. In addition to the

MAP

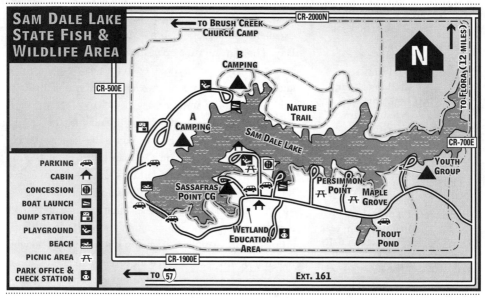

SAM DALE LAKE STATE FISH & WILDLIFE AREA

CR-2000N

TO BRUSH CREEK CHURCH CAMP

N

TO FLORA (12 MILES)

CR-500E

B CAMPING

NATURE TRAIL

A CAMPING

Sam Dale Lake

CR-700E

YOUTH GROUP

PERSIMMON POINT

SASSAFRAS POINT CG

MAPLE GROVE

WETLAND EDUCATION AREA

TROUT POND

CR-1900E

TO 57

EXT. 161

PARKING
CABIN
CONCESSION
BOAT LAUNCH
DUMP STATION
PLAYGROUND
BEACH
PICNIC AREA
PARK OFFICE & CHECK STATION

MAP

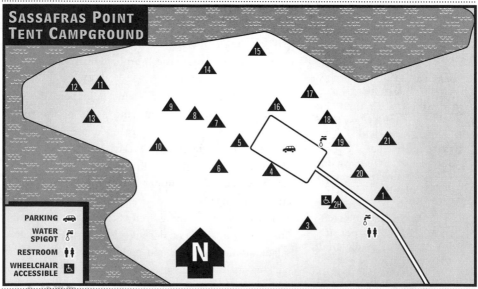

SASSAFRAS POINT TENT CAMPGROUND

15

14

12 11

9

13

8 7

16

17

18

10

5

19

21

6

4

20

1

2H

3

N

PARKING
WATER SPIGOT
RESTROOM
WHEELCHAIR ACCESSIBLE

usual central Illinois species, such as catfish, bullhead, largemouth bass, crappie, bluegill, and even a few muskie, you can fish for rainbow trout in Trout Pond: it is one of 43 sites the IDNR stocks twice a year with this delicacy. Trout seasons open the first Saturday in April and the third Saturday in October, and a special trout stamp is necessary in addition to the regular Illinois fishing license.

GETTING THERE

From Salem, take I-57 south to Exit 109. Go east on IL 161 about 22 miles to the large brown sign on the left for Sam Dale Lake. Turn left onto CR 700 East and drive 0.8 miles to the park entrance, on the left.

From IL 45 in Cisne, drive 7.2 miles west on IL 161 and make a right onto CR 700 East to reach the park entrance, on the left.

GPS COORDINATES

UTM Zone 16S
Easting 0363561
Northing 4266520
Latitude N 38° 32' 11.8797"
Longitude W 88° 33' 55.6323"

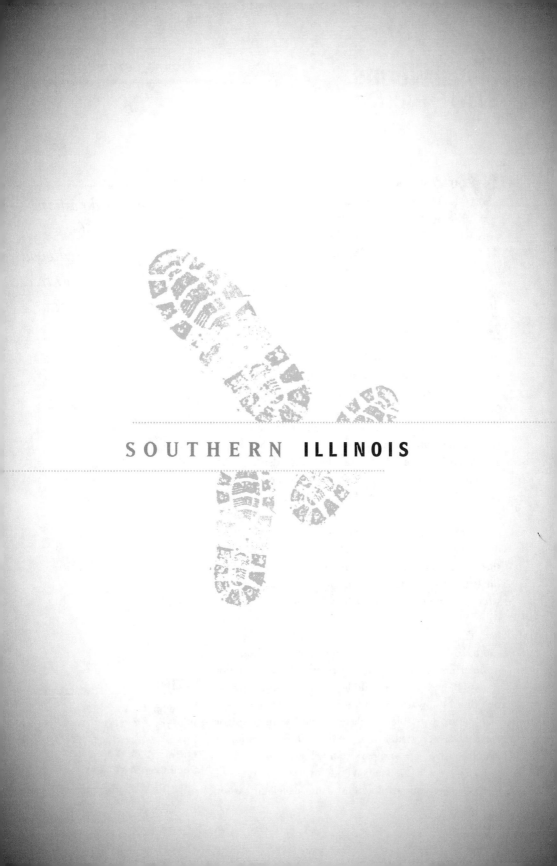

SOUTHERN ILLINOIS

30
BEALL WOODS STATE PARK

YOU CAN VISIT DICKSON MOUNDS, Cahokia Mounds, Millstone Bluff, and other places in Illinois to view artifacts of the Native Americans who lived here long before Europeans came. At Beall (pronounced "bell") Woods State Park, however, you can see what the woodlands themselves looked like in those pre-pioneer days. Within the 635 acres of this park on the banks of the Wabash River are 329 acres of old-growth woods—virtually untouched by man—the largest remnant of the original deciduous forests that once covered perhaps 40 percent of the state. In this Midwestern equivalent of California's redwood forest, some 300 trees grow to more than 120 feet tall.

For the sake of the centuries-old trees, however, you cannot camp in the woods. The campground is a simple half loop of 16 sites, set along the edge of a flat open field near the park's entrance. A line of trees stands behind the sites to the west, but there isn't a lot of shade where you camp. I wouldn't call it scenic, but there's plenty of space, it's clean, and it's not real busy outside of holidays. On an average weekend perhaps four or five sites will be occupied. There's room for RVs to park, but since there's no electricity or showers, you probably won't see more than the occasional pop-up camper.

As you enter the park, the campground is on the left. The campground road is one-way, from north to south, so head past the southern end to enter from the north. I prefer the sites on the right, outside the loop; sites 6, 8, and 9, in the middle, are even more spread out. Site 14, toward the end, is nicely shaded. Each site has one or two tables; vault toilets and a water spigot are centrally located, across from site 9. Registration is simple—just set up, and park staff will come by later.

You come to Beall Woods to see the trees, of course. Start your exploration at the excellent visitor

> *In this Midwestern equivalent of California's redwood forest, some 300 trees grow to more than 120 feet tall.*

RATINGS

Beauty: ✩ ✩
Privacy: ✩ ✩ ✩
Spaciousness: ✩ ✩ ✩
Quiet: ✩ ✩ ✩
Security: ✩ ✩ ✩ ✩
Cleanliness: ✩ ✩ ✩ ✩ ✩

ADDRESS:	9285 Beall Woods Avenue, Mount Carmel, IL 62863
OPERATED BY:	IDNR
CONTACT:	(618) 298-2442, www.dnr.state.il .us/lands/land mgt/parks/r5/ beall.htm
OPEN:	Year-round
SITES:	Class C: 16
EACH SITE:	Picnic table, ground grill
ASSIGNMENT:	First come, first served
REGISTRATION:	Set up, and park personnel will come by
FACILITIES:	Water spigots, vault toilets
PARKING:	At site
FEE:	$8 per night
ELEVATION:	407 feet
RESTRICTIONS:	*Pets:* On leash only *Fires:* In fire rings only *Alcohol:* Not permitted *Vehicles:* 2 per site *Other:* 14-day limit; 1 RV and 1 tent, or 2 tents per site; 4 adults or 1 family per site

center, where you can pick up a trail map and see the interactive exhibits on the history and ecology of the area. This is a kid-friendly place—many school groups come here each year for environmental education programs. Additionally, the site interpreter leads a variety of free nature hikes and activities, some especially for kids and requiring advance registration. Check the Web site for scheduled activities. The visitor center is open Sunday and Monday from noon to 4 p.m., and from 8 a.m. to 4 p.m. the rest of the week.

Five loop trails, totaling 6.25 miles, wander through the woods, along Coffee and Sugar creeks, and by the wide Wabash River. This portion of Beall Woods is an Illinois Nature Preserve and a federally designated national landmark, so pets, bicycles, and horses are not allowed, and hikers should stay on the established trails to protect the natural resources (and avoid the large patches of poison ivy). The trails are easy to hike and well marked—the only hazard is that you could walk into a ravine as you're gawking at the trees overhead. Of the 64 species of trees in the park, 4—the black gum (104 feet), sugarberry (120 feet), shellbark hickory (127 feet), and mockernut hickory (122 feet)—have their state champions at Beall Woods. Hundreds of others, while not the tallest of their species, reach awe-inspiring height and girth. (For a complete list of Illinois' largest trees by species, and the GPS locations for some, check **web.extension.uiuc.edu/forestry/ibtr08_mar03.pdf.** And in case you absolutely have to know—as I did—the tallest tree in the state is a 165-foot red oak in Dixon Springs State Park.)

Two trails begin just behind the visitor center. The 1-mile Tuliptree Trail is the easiest, circling through upland woods and along a small bluff over Coffee Creek. White Oak Trail is 1.25 miles—moderately easy, with a couple flights of steps—and is one of the best for viewing the large trees. From the southern tip of White Oak you can cross a bridge over Coffee Creek to access the 1.75-mile Ridgway Trail, which passes through a reforested field along the Wabash River. The connected 0.5-mile Sweet Gum and 1.75-mile Schenck trails are north of Coffee Creek. You can reach them by crossing Rocky Ford, 0.3 miles north of the visitor center (plan

MAP

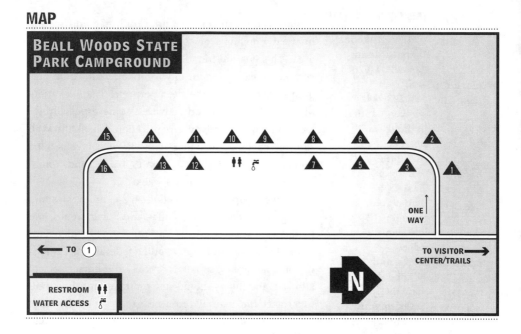

BEALL WOODS STATE PARK CAMPGROUND

15 14 11 10 9 8 6 4 2

16 13 12 7 5 3 1

ONE WAY

← TO ①

TO VISITOR → CENTER/TRAILS

N

RESTROOM
WATER ACCESS

to get your feet wet), or you can access them from a separate parking lot north of the main entrance: Exit the park, turn right, then immediately make another right onto CR 800 East; proceed 1.3 miles north to the lot on the right as the road curves left. Note that the Ridgway, Sweet Gum, and Schenck trails are closed when flooded.

Beall Woods also has a 15-acre lake where you can fish for bluegill, largemouth bass, and catfish and is among 43 in the state stocked with trout each spring and fall. The park occasionally hosts scout camping events and often welcomes school groups for day visits. These are always scheduled in advance, so if you want to camp (or just hike) in peace, I recommend calling first to find out if any large groups are on the calendar.

GETTING THERE

From I-64 at Exit 130, take IL 1 north 12 miles to Keensburg. Turn right on First Street (CR 16), then go 1 block to Market Street (CR 3) and turn left. Follow the road as it curves left and becomes CR 900 North; it's 2 miles to Beall Woods. From US 50 at IL 1 in Lawrenceville, take IL 1 south 33 miles to Keensburg. Turn left on First Street and proceed as above.

GPS COORDINATES

UTM Zone 16S
Easting 0427048
Northing 4244744
Latitude N 38° 20' 52.3624"
Longitude W 87° 50' 5.5010"

31
RANDOLPH COUNTY STATE FISH & WILDLIFE AREA

> *This underappreciated camping getaway is neither too busy nor too far from some unique natural venues.*

RANDOLPH COUNTY STATE FISH & WILDLIFE Area is another of the underappreciated camping getaways in southern Illinois; it's neither too busy nor too far from some unique natural venues. Among the three campgrounds, the one with electric hookups draws most of the traffic, leaving the other two, which are less popular, available for tent campers.

Enter the park, arrive at a T-intersection, and turn right. The next left brings you into Oak Ridge, the smallest and least-used of Randolph County's three campgrounds. There are supposed to be 15 unnumbered sites here, but from the ground grills and tables, I'd say there are 12. Regardless, you can set up near any grill and move tables around as needed. Just park on the grass near your site. All these are good choices—site 9 is great for shade.

For a more scenic option, check out the two walk-in sites down by the lake. You can park in the loop past sites 11 and 12 to unload, and carry your gear down the steps to the lakefront, about 200 feet. These are set apart from the other sites (up the hill), but be aware that those campers may come down to fish.

Down the road from the Oak Ridge entrance is the park office, where you register, and the Pine Ridge RV campground—it has been recently renovated, but pass it up for tent camping. Head back north on the main park road, go past the road to the group campground, and take the next left to Rolling Hills Campground. Again, these sites are unnumbered; there are supposed to be 31, but I count 25. The sites are spread along the road and in two small loops to the north, each with a parking lot (though you can pull right up to each site). The sites on the first loop, 1 through 6 on my map, have poor shade. Those at the far end of the second loop, sites 11 through 13, are more spacious and shaded. My other favorite is the last drive-in site, number 25.

RATINGS

Beauty: ✿ ✿ ✿
Privacy: ✿ ✿ ✿
Spaciousness: ✿ ✿ ✿
Quiet: ✿ ✿ ✿ ✿
Security: ✿ ✿ ✿ ✿
Cleanliness: ✿ ✿ ✿ ✿ ✿

If the campground is busy and you'd like a little more space, the walk-in sites at the end of the Rolling Hills road are a good choice. The first is conveniently close to the walk-in parking and is well shaded. I prefer the second, about 100 feet down the trail. The third is another 170 feet and not worth the additional steps.

Fishing is popular here, and the clear lake is stocked with channel catfish, redear, bluegill, walleye, saugeye, and rainbow trout. While some sources mention a concession, it hasn't operated for several years. You can still rent boats from the park office—$10 for a boat, oars, and lifejackets for the whole day; $20 more gets you a battery and trolling motor.

Just a few miles (as the crow flies) southwest of Randolph County is Piney Creek Ravine State Natural Area, a fascinating hiking destination, which contains the largest body of prehistoric rock art in Illinois. A fairly rugged 2.5-mile loop, the hike is nicest in the spring, when the creek and waterfalls are flowing.

From the park, go west 1 mile to Palestine Road, then make a left and drive 3.8 miles south to Van Zant Street in Chester, then take a left and make a right onto SR 3. Turn left (south) and go 11.5 miles to Hog Hill Road, where you'll see a brown Piney Creek sign. Turn left, drive 3.8 miles to a T-intersection, then make a right; the next left will put you on Rock Crusher Road. Go 1 mile to Piney Creek Road, then take a left and travel 1.6 miles to the parking area, on the left. Pick up the trail to the left of the parking area, between two fencerows. Hike a short distance to the grassy area on the right, and cross to the preserve entrance. Be careful as you cross the slippery wet sandstone streambed.

Randolph County is about 40 miles from Illinois Caverns State Natural Area, one of the most interesting geological wonders of southern Illinois. Illinois Caverns is the state's third-longest cave, with 6 miles of passageways containing canyons, beautiful formations, small waterfalls, and the occasional bat or salamander. This is not a tourist cave, however. There are no paved walkways, lights, or guided tours. You should plan on (and dress for) walking through cold 55° water and getting dirty. Hiking the main passage is comparable to hiking

KEY INFORMATION

ADDRESS:	4301 South Lake Drive, Chester, IL 62233
OPERATED BY:	IDNR
CONTACT:	(618) 826-2706, www.dnr.state.il .us/lands/land mgt/parks/r4/ rand.htm
OPEN:	Year-round
SITES:	Class C: 37 vehicle-access sites; Class D: 5 walk-in sites; Class B: 105 electric sites
EACH SITE:	Picnic table, ground grill
ASSIGNMENT:	First come, first served
REGISTRATION:	Come to office first to register
FACILITIES:	Water spigots, vault toilets
PARKING:	At site (Class B & C); in lot (Class D)
FEE:	Class B: $18 per night; Class C: $8 per night; Class D: $6 per night
ELEVATION:	510 feet
RESTRICTIONS:	*Pets:* On leash only *Fires:* In fire rings only *Alcohol:* Permitted *Vehicles:* 2 per site *Other:* 14-day limit; 1 RV and 1 tent, or 2 tents per site; 6 people per site

MAP

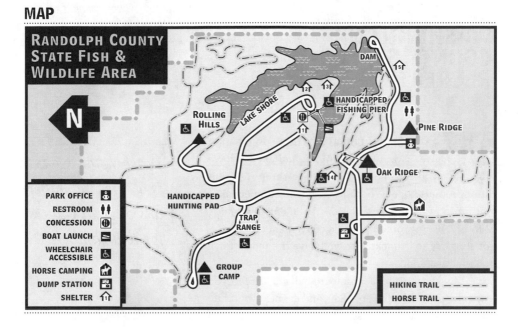

RANDOLPH COUNTY STATE FISH & WILDLIFE AREA

N

DAM

HANDICAPPED FISHING PIER

ROLLING HILLS

LAKE SHORE

PINE RIDGE

OAK RIDGE

PARK OFFICE
RESTROOM
CONCESSION
BOAT LAUNCH
WHEELCHAIR ACCESSIBLE
HORSE CAMPING
DUMP STATION
SHELTER

HANDICAPPED HUNTING PAD

TRAP RANGE

GROUP CAMP

HIKING TRAIL —————
HORSE TRAIL —·—·—·—

GETTING THERE

From the north, take IL 3 south 2.5 miles past Ellis Grove, to Shawneetown Trail. Turn left, go 3.6 miles east to Palestine Road. Turn right, go 1.6 miles, then make a left at the park entrance.

From the south, take IL 3 north to Chester. Turn right on State Street, go 0.3 miles to Van Zant Street, turn left, drive 0.25 miles to Palestine Road, and turn right. Travel 3.8 miles, then make a right at the park entrance.

GPS COORDINATES

UTM Zone 16S
Easting 0253583
Northing 4206416
Latitude N 37° 58' 19.0215"
Longitude W 89° 48' 19.1130"

a rocky canyon, but there are plenty of side passages to explore where crawling is the only way forward.

There is no charge, but you must fill out a permit form before entering the cave and have at least four people in your group, three sources of light per person, hard hats, and sturdy shoes with a good tread. I recommend a helmet headlamp, freeing your hands to help you climb and crawl; also bring along drinking water, a snack, and a complete change of clothes. (There are changing rooms above ground.) Illinois Caverns is currently open Thursday through Saturday from 8:30 a.m. to 2:30 p.m. Check the Web site **www.dnr.state.il.us/lands/landmgt/parks/r4/ caverns/index.htm** for complete details.

To get there, drive 29 miles north of Chester on IL 3 to Kaskaskia Road—watch for the small brown Illinois Caverns sign on the left. Turn left, go 2 miles into the little town of Burksville, and turn left at the Illinois Caverns sign onto KK Road. Go 1 mile to G Road, turn right, and travel 2 miles south. Illinois Caverns is on the right.

WASHINGTON COUNTY STATE Recreation Area is kind of a camping buffet—you have a lot of choices. There are three different campgrounds, two especially for tent campers and one with walk-in sites. Throw in a 258-acre lake, showers, fishing, boating, and a convenient concession for supplies and snacks, and you have the recipe for a relaxing weekend.

Little Bear is the first campground you'll see as you enter the park—take the first right, and the next left. Little Bear consists of a single road with a loop at the end; stairs lead down to the lake and a fishing dock. It's a pretty, wooded, grassy area, with 20 unnumbered sites (I numbered them on my map to make it easy). Most sites offer plenty of room, and those on the right as you drive in (sites 1 through 7) are a bit farther apart. If you want to be close the lake, sites 6 and 8 at the end are good—you can pop down the stairs to fish any time of the day or night. Site 12 has a small picnic pavilion next to it, which is great if it rains. The only sites I didn't like were 7, 10, and 11 (too small and sloping), and 19 and 20 (too close to the road). You won't see any gravel parking spots, but you're welcome to park on the grass next to your site.

Note that youth groups frequent Little Bear. However, before you panic, thinking you might be overrun by a herd of Boy Scouts at midnight, know that groups have to make advance arrangements, and the sign at the entrance to the campground will indicate if it's been reserved for a group that day.

The next campground is Lonely Oaks—take the second right after the park entrance, then hang a left at the crossroads. Lonely Oaks has 32 unnumbered vehicle-access sites along three prongs of a branching road, plus 5 walk-in sites. Site 6, on the right as you enter, is great, being well away from the road and shaded. Site 15, at the end of the middle fork, is in its

> *Washington County is a camping buffet—lots of great choices for tent campers.*

RATINGS

Beauty: ✪ ✪ ✪ ✪
Privacy: ✪ ✪ ✪
Spaciousness: ✪ ✪ ✪ ✪ ✪
Quiet: ✪ ✪ ✪ ✪
Security: ✪ ✪ ✪ ✪
Cleanliness: ✪ ✪ ✪ ✪ ✪

ADDRESS:	18500 Conservation Drive, Nashville, IL 62263
OPERATED BY:	IDNR
CONTACT:	(618) 327-3137, www.dnr.state.il.us/lands/land mgt/parks/r4/washco.htm
OPEN:	Year-round
SITES:	Class C: 52 non-electric sites and 16 walk-in sites; Class A: 51 electric sites; 1 cabin
EACH SITE:	Picnic table, fire ring or ground grill; electric in Class A only
ASSIGNMENT:	First come, first served
REGISTRATION:	Register at the office or park staff will come by
FACILITIES:	Water spigots, vault toilets, shower house
PARKING:	At site (Class A and some Class C); in lot (walk-in)
FEE:	Class A: $20 per night, $30 per night holidays; Class C: $8 per night; $40 per night for cabin, plus $5 reservation fee
ELEVATION:	499 feet
RESTRICTIONS:	*Pets:* On leash only *Fires:* In fire rings only *Alcohol:* Permitted *Vehicles:* 2 per site *Other:* 14-day limit; 1 RV and 1 tent, or 2 tents per site; 4 adults or 1 family per site

own little wooded nook, and site 20 is on a flat, grassy area over the hill and next to the stairs leading down to the lake and fishing dock. Site 29, at the end of the left fork, offers a great view of the lake. Only the sites in the middle (18, 19, and 21 through 24) seem cramped and open. I camped at one of the walk-in sites at the end of the right fork and loved it. It's just a short walk from the parking lot (300 feet at most), and though there were others in the campground, I felt like I had the place to myself. As at Little Bear, you can park on the grass (except at the walk-in sites).

North of Lonely Oaks is the third campground, Shady Rest, with a single loop of 51 electric sites. The clean, excellent shower house is located at the entrance and open to all campers from April 1 to October 31. Surprisingly, at the end the loop there's also a parking lot and 11 walk-in tent sites. Five sites are right by the lot, but the other six are spread through the woods on a point overlooking the lake. For the best view, head to the one farthest out. Nearby is the park's only rental cabin, which has heat and air-conditioning, a table and chairs, beds for six, and a grill. This is a great combination if you have some family members who want a roof over their heads (like mom and dad), and others who want to tent camp nearby (like the kids). (Be sure to reserve the cabin well in advance.)

Which campground to pick? Little Bear is smaller and more wooded, Lonely Oaks is more spread out, and the tent sites in Shady Rest are within walking distance of the showers. The electric sites at Shady Rest fill up most good weekends, but the tent areas are usually no more than half full outside of holidays. So browse the options, pick a site, and settle in. Park staff will come by later to register you.

The boat docks and park concession are south of Little Bear campground. There you can purchase ice, firewood, fishing tackle, bait, soft drinks, sandwiches, and snacks. If you'd like to explore the lake, you can rent kayaks or johnboats, with or without a motor. The concession is open daily April 1 to November 1 from 7 a.m. to 7 p.m.

Washington County Recreation Area has one official hiking trail, a 7-mile loop that circles the lake.

MAP

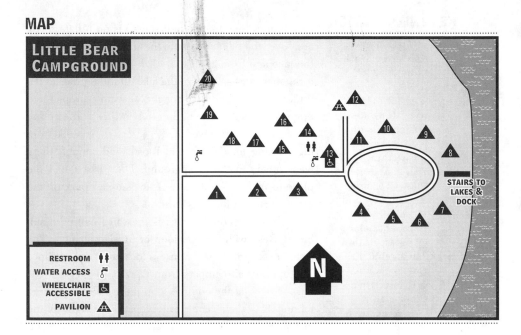

LITTLE BEAR CAMPGROUND

STAIRS TO LAKES & DOCK

N

RESTROOM 👫
WATER ACCESS 🚰
WHEELCHAIR ACCESSIBLE ♿
PAVILION ⛺

MAP

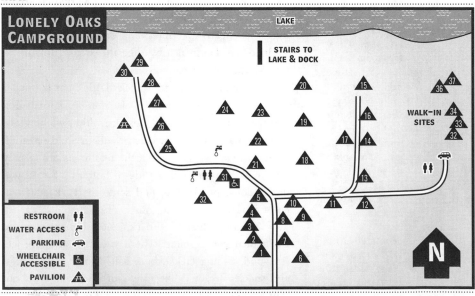

LONELY OAKS CAMPGROUND

LAKE

STAIRS TO LAKE & DOCK

WALK-IN SITES

N

RESTROOM 👫
WATER ACCESS 🚰
PARKING 🚗
WHEELCHAIR ACCESSIBLE ♿
PAVILION ⛺

Two-thirds of the loop follows the park road; the remaining wooded trail is rarely hiked and challenging to follow. The road portion is worth hiking or driving, though, as it passes through the woods on the eastern side of the lake, which most park visitors don't see. This is the best area for wildlife viewing, and the trees are beautiful in the fall.

GETTING THERE

From I-64, take Exit 50 and go south 7.5 miles on IL 127 through Nashville to Conservation Drive. Turn left and drive 1 mile to the park entrance.

GPS COORDINATES

UTM Zone 16S
Easting 0293543
Northing 4239551
Latitude N 38° 16' 49.0878"
Longitude W 89° 21' 37.3399"

IF YOU LIKE TO CAMP in places not quite so tame, Pyramid State Park might be for you. With more than 19,000 acres, Pyramid is Illinois' largest state park, almost all of it on land that was once strip-mined for coal. Time and man's intervention have restored the land to a haven for wildlife, a rugged mix of heavily forested hills, meadows, wetlands, and dozens of small lakes. Hunters, fishermen, hikers, and campers can all find plenty of room to get away.

Most visitors will spend their time in what's called the "Original Pyramid," the 3,200 acres first designated as a state park in 1968. That's where you'll find the park office and three primitive campgrounds with 48 total sites, plus about 11 hike-in campsites. All sites have a picnic table and ground grill, and each campground has vault toilets. The only water spigot is located at the park office, by the entrance. Most of the vehicular access sites are small, though there are some lakeside gems among them. Outside of archery season (October 1 to mid-January), Pyramid sees very few campers—and even then, less than a quarter of sites will be occupied on the busiest weekend.

As you enter Pyramid, take the first left at the office (where you'll return to register) and go straight back to Heron Campground. Heron has nine sites laid out in a row along the north side of the road, with a fence and croplands to the south. These sites are flat and grassy, with woods behind and trees around, providing plenty of shade. Though not widely separated, as a group these are the largest pull-in campsites at Pyramid. I like site 2 because it's set back from the road a bit. Pyramid doesn't draw many RVs because there's no electricity or water hookups, but Heron is the one campground where you may occasionally see a small pop-up or trailer.

To get to Boulder Lake Campground, turn left out of Heron, go north, and turn right at the T-junction.

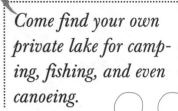

Come find your own private lake for camping, fishing, and even canoeing.

RATINGS

Beauty: ✿ ✿ ✿
Privacy: ✿ ✿ ✿ ✿ ✿
Spaciousness: ✿ ✿ ✿
Quiet: ✿ ✿ ✿ ✿ ✿
Security: ✿ ✿ ✿ ✿
Cleanliness: ✿ ✿ ✿ ✿ ✿

KEY INFORMATION

ADDRESS: 1562 Pyramid Park Road, Pinckneyville, IL

OPERATED BY: IDNR

CONTACT: (618) 357-2574, www.dnr.state.il.us/lands/landmgt/parks/r5/pyramid.htm

OPEN: Year-round

SITES: Class C: 48 sites; Class D: 11 hike-in sites

EACH SITE: Table, ground grill

ASSIGNMENT: First come, first served

REGISTRATION: Register at the office or at self-registration post if office is closed

FACILITIES: Water spigot (at office only), vault toilets

PARKING: At campsite; at nearest parking lot for hike-in sites

FEE: Class C: $8 per tent; hike-in sites: $6 per night

ELEVATION: 410 feet

RESTRICTIONS: *Pets:* On leash only
Fires: In fire rings only
Alcohol: Permitted
Vehicles: 2 per site
Other: 14-day limit; 2 tents or 1 RV per site; 4 adults or 1 family per site

The road ends at the campground, with sites 1 to 9 to the left and 10 to 18 to the right. Site 1, at the north end, is right on Boulder Lake and next to the boat ramp, and site 11 offers the most space and a bit of seclusion, with some surrounding brush and trees. Sites 2 through 10, 17, and 18 are tiny and too close together. The small field and grove of trees past site 14 at the south end contains eight sites for equestrians only.

The North Campground at Pyramid is on the opposite side of the park. From the entrance, go straight past the office and follow the road all the way to the northeast corner, where the campground with 19 sites is tucked between five small lakes. The better sites are located at either end of the campground road, next to the lakes. To the right (east), sites 21, 22, and 23 are small, but in a very pretty spot by themselves on Clear Lake. If no one else is camping nearby, 23, in particular, is a good choice. At the west end (to the left), sites 4 and 5, and 7 through 11 are good, situated between Beehive and Plum lakes. Site 5 is perched atop a small hill by itself, and site 7 is my favorite, fairly large, right on Beehive Lake and near a small fishing dock. (Sites 1, 2, 3, and 6 seem to have disappeared.) The sites in the middle are too small and close together.

If you want real seclusion and don't mind walking a bit, Pyramid has 11 separate hike-in sites, ranging from 200 yards to 1 mile from the nearest parking lot. Several are right on the water, so with a little effort you can have your own private lake for camping, fishing, and canoeing. There is a beautiful site on Hook Lake, about a 0.5 miles from the nearest lot. To get there, go north past the office and the archery range to the parking area on the curve. From there take the trail heading downhill to the west. You'll find one site along the trail at about 0.4 miles, but continue another 500 feet to the one on the lake. Most of the hike-in sites have a table, ground grill, and trashcan. Note that not all the hike-in sites on older park maps are currently maintained. Check in at the office before camping, both to register and to find out which sites are usable and where to park for easiest access.

The 16.5 miles of trails at Pyramid are wide and well maintained and are open to hikers, equestrians,

MAP

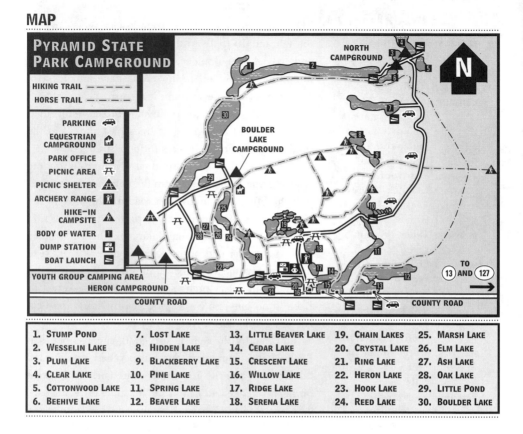

PYRAMID STATE PARK CAMPGROUND

| HIKING TRAIL | – – – – – |
| HORSE TRAIL | – · – · – |

PARKING	
EQUESTRIAN CAMPGROUND	
PARK OFFICE	
PICNIC AREA	
PICNIC SHELTER	
ARCHERY RANGE	
HIKE–IN CAMPSITE	
BODY OF WATER	
DUMP STATION	
BOAT LAUNCH	

YOUTH GROUP CAMPING AREA
HERON CAMPGROUND

COUNTY ROAD   COUNTY ROAD

NORTH CAMPGROUND

BOULDER LAKE CAMPGROUND

N

TO ⑬ AND ⑫⑦

1. STUMP POND	7. LOST LAKE	13. LITTLE BEAVER LAKE	19. CHAIN LAKES	25. MARSH LAKE
2. WESSELIN LAKE	8. HIDDEN LAKE	14. CEDAR LAKE	20. CRYSTAL LAKE	26. ELM LAKE
3. PLUM LAKE	9. BLACKBERRY LAKE	15. CRESCENT LAKE	21. RING LAKE	27. ASH LAKE
4. CLEAR LAKE	10. PINE LAKE	16. WILLOW LAKE	22. HERON LAKE	28. OAK LAKE
5. COTTONWOOD LAKE	11. SPRING LAKE	17. RIDGE LAKE	23. HOOK LAKE	29. LITTLE POND
6. BEEHIVE LAKE	12. BEAVER LAKE	18. SERENA LAKE	24. REED LAKE	30. BOULDER LAKE

and even mountain bikers. Pyramid attracts plenty of wildlife, and you're likely to see deer, wild turkey, migrating waterfowl (in season)—and ticks. When I was there in the spring, ticks weren't noticeable at the campgrounds, but I picked up quite a collection hiking the trails. Take the necessary precautions, or plan to camp in the fall when they're not as prevalent.

GPS COORDINATES

UTM Zone 16S
Easting 0287837
Northing 4209069
Latitude N 38° 0' 16.1731"
Longitude W 89° 24' 59.3287"

GETTING THERE

From US 51 in DuQuoin, head 9.6 miles west on IL 152 (Main Street, which becomes Pyatt-Cutler Road at 6.8 miles) to the park entrance, on the left. From the junction of IL 154 and IL 13 in Pinckneyville (Main and Water streets), go 5.5 miles south on IL 13 to Pyatt-Cutler Road. Turn right and drive 2.5 miles to the park entrance on the left.

34
WAYNE FITZGERRELL STATE PARK

> *This ideal little tent campground lies amid a big outdoor recreational mecca.*

IF YOU SEARCH THE WEB for "Rend Lake" in south-central Illinois, you'll find a resort, a golf course, a college, a marina, and several large and usually crowded RV campgrounds. It doesn't sound like the kind of place for a frugal tent camper hunting for more nature and fewer people. However, Wayne Fitzgerrell State Park offers an ideal little walk-in tent campground on a shaded point projecting into the lake. You'll rarely find solitude there, but you can camp in relative peace and still take advantage of all the lake has to offer.

Wayne Fitzgerrell is part of the huge outdoor mecca surrounding the 19,000-acre Rend Lake, managed jointly by the Illinois Department of Natural Resources, the U.S. Army Corps of Engineers, and the Rend Lake Conservancy. The park includes an enormous 243-site RV campground, but the walk-in tent area is all by itself to the north. In fact, it's far enough from the main campground and resort that no one comes through except tent campers, and close enough that you can drive to all the amenities and recreational options available.

As you enter the park from the south, drive 3 miles north to just past the impressive Rend Lake Resort. Turn right, go 0.5 miles, then make a left at the sign for tent camping. This road dead-ends at the loop, where you can park and walk to any of the 17 tent sites spread around the grassy point. In the middle of the loop you'll find the single water spigot, and the vault toilets to one side. Each site has a table and a ground grill.

Most of the sites are well shaded and fairly far apart. Since this little campground will be busy most weekends, I suggest heading for the sites farthest out, so other campers won't be walking through or around your site to get to theirs. If you don't want to carry your gear far, try site 1, 2, or 3 to the east—they're far enough from

RATINGS

Beauty: ✪ ✪ ✪ ✪
Privacy: ✪ ✪ ✪
Spaciousness: ✪ ✪ ✪
Quiet: ✪ ✪ ✪ ✪
Security: ✪ ✪ ✪ ✪
Cleanliness: ✪ ✪ ✪ ✪

the lot to give you some privacy, and there are no other sites behind them. However I highly recommend heading away from the lot to the end of the point. Sites 6, 7, 8, 14, and 15 are closest to the lakeshore and offer beautiful views—you can watch the sun set to the west. Sites 14 and 15 are sunny; 6, 7, and 8 are more shaded. Just set up and park personnel will come by to register you. Note that the walk-in campground fees do not include use of the shower houses in the main campground.

If your easily bored kids (or you) prefer lots of activity to just sitting around the campsite, the Rend Lake area offers so much that you could all be exhausted by nightfall. Fishing, boating, and hunting are, of course, popular, but you can also enjoy swimming, waterskiing, hiking, mountain biking, horseback riding, golf, and trap-shooting, or else visit an art museum, winery, and shops. Since the lake is large and the facilities spread out, scope out the options online in advance **www.mvs.usace.army.mil/rend, www.rendlake.com,** and **www.rendlakeresort.com.**

A good place to start at Rend Lake is the visitor center at the south end, on the east side of the dam. There you'll find not only current information but also exhibits on the area, a 250-gallon aquarium featuring Rend Lake species, and a terrarium of live snakes. Starting in 2009, the center will open every day from April 1 to October 31 from 10 a.m. to 5 p.m. From Wayne Fitzgerrell, go south through the park to IL 154, turn right, and continue across the lake to Rend City Road. Turn left, head south about 6 miles to reach Rend Lake Dam Road, and turn left again.

At the resort, you can rent pontoon boats, paddleboats, or mouse boats (think "miniature ski boat") from the shop by the tennis courts. You can also purchase ice, firewood, snacks, groceries, and camping and fishing supplies there, as well as rent mountain bikes. About 4.5 miles of level, easy bike trail extend from Rend Lake College to the north, through the resort, and along the eastern shore south to the park office. After a full day of activity, you can avoid campfire cooking and splurge a bit at the resort's excellent Windows Restaurant, where you can get just about anything from lobster and prime rib to grilled cheese.

KEY INFORMATION

ADDRESS:	11094 Ranger Road, Whittington, IL 62897
OPERATED BY:	IDNR
CONTACT:	(618) 629-2320, www.dnr.state.il .us/lands/land mgt/parks/r5/ wayne.htm
OPEN:	Year-round
SITES:	Class C: 17 walk-in tent sites, Class A: 243 electric sites
EACH SITE:	Electric in Class A only; picnic table, ground grill
ASSIGNMENT:	First come, first served
REGISTRATION:	Set up and park personnel will come by for Class C; register with host for Class A
FACILITIES:	Water spigots, vault toilets; showers for Class A only
PARKING:	At site (Class A); in lot (Class C)
FEE:	Class A: $20 per night, $30 per night holidays; Class C: $6 per night
ELEVATION:	417 feet
RESTRICTIONS:	*Pets:* On leash only *Fires:* In fire rings only *Alcohol:* Permitted *Vehicles:* 2 per site *Other:* 14-day limit; 1 RV and 1 tent, or 2 tents per site; 4 adults or 1 family per site

MAP

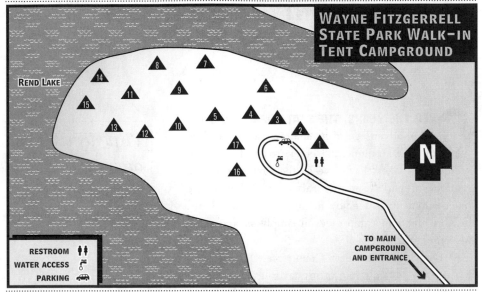

WAYNE FITZGERRELL STATE PARK WALK-IN TENT CAMPGROUND

REND LAKE

N

RESTROOM
WATER ACCESS
PARKING

TO MAIN
CAMPGROUND
AND ENTRANCE

GETTING THERE

From I-57, take Exit 77 to
IL 154 and head west 2 miles
to the park entrance,
on the right.

GPS COORDINATES

UTM Zone 16S
Easting 0329187
Northing 4217547
Latitude N 38° 5' 22.5457"
Longitude W 88° 56' 51.2"

Swimming is available at the spacious South Sandusky beach on the west side of the lake, managed by the Corps of Engineers. (The North Marcum beach, which you may see advertised in older brochures, is no longer open for swimming.) The beach costs $1 per person over 12 years of age per day, with the maximum charge $4 per vehicle. You can take advantage of the hot showers and changing facilities there, too. To reach it from the campground, cross the lake on IL 154 and head south on Rend City Road about 3.25 miles to the South Sandusky entrance.

Nine miles of equestrian trails also loop through the park. Previously, a concessionaire offered horseback riding as well as mule-drawn wagon rides, but as of mid-2008 they had closed.

35
HAMILTON COUNTY STATE FISH & WILDLIFE AREA

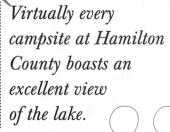

> *Virtually every campsite at Hamilton County boasts an excellent view of the lake.*

OVER THE YEARS, THE STATE OF ILLINOIS has taken advantage of its shallow valleys, rolling hills, and innumerable creeks to construct small recreational lakes that serve as the centerpiece of a number of parks and natural areas. I love these places—sometimes I enjoy fishing, but mostly I just love to hike and camp or even simply sit and relax near the open water.

Of all these, Hamilton County State Fish & Wildlife Area is certainly one of my favorites. The lake is beautiful, and the staff and campground hosts are friendly and helpful. You can fish or hike a few short trails, but most visitors come just to relax. Best of all, the campground is perfectly positioned on a wide point jutting into Dolan Lake and has been laid out so that virtually every site has an excellent view of the lake, which borders the campground on three sides. The tall trees throughout provide ample shade yet leave it feeling open and airy.

As you enter Hamilton County off IL 14, turn left and follow the signs south to the Piney Wood camping area. The main campground entrance will be on the left; just past it on the right is a small parking area followed by four cabins. Park here to access the ten walk-in sites, just to the west. These are great for tent campers—just enough of a walk to keep them underutilized but still readily accessible and close to the main campground's excellent facilities.

Walk down a little dip and back up, and site 1 is on the left. If it isn't already taken, this is my first choice—spacious, airy, and well shaded, with a gorgeous view of the lake, and just 300 feet from the parking lot. A bit farther down the trail are sites 2 and 3, which face each other and thus are a bit too neighborly. Site 4 is off by itself, 450 feet from parking, and is comfortably situated under tall pine trees. Site 5 is in a clearing to

RATINGS

Beauty: ☆ ☆ ☆ ☆ ☆
Privacy: ☆ ☆ ☆ ☆
Spaciousness: ☆ ☆ ☆
Quiet: ☆ ☆ ☆ ☆
Security: ☆ ☆ ☆ ☆ ☆
Cleanliness: ☆ ☆ ☆ ☆ ☆

ADDRESS:	RR 4, Box 242, McLeansboro, IL
OPERATED BY:	IDNR
CONTACT:	(618) 773-4340, www.dnr.state.il .us/lands/land mgt/parks/r5/ hamilton.htm
OPEN:	Year-round
SITES:	Class C: 10 walk-in sites; Class A: 60 sites; 4 cabins
EACH SITE:	Picnic table, ground grill; electric (Class A only)
ASSIGNMENT:	First come, first served; cabins reservable
REGISTRATION:	Register with campground host (if available) or at the office
FACILITIES:	Water spigots, vault toilets, shower house (closed late Dec.–Mar.)
PARKING:	At site (Class A); in lot (Class C)
FEE:	Class A: $20 per night, $30 per night holidays; Class C: $8 per night; cabin: $45 per night; $5 reservation fee
ELEVATION:	459 feet
RESTRICTIONS:	*Pets:* On leash only *Fires:* In fire rings only *Alcohol:* Permitted *Vehicles:* 2 per site *Other:* 14-day limit; 1 camping unit (RV or tent) or 2 smaller tents per site; 4 adults or 1 family of 6 per site

the right but is a bit too close to the trail, and sites 6 and 7 are a bit farther down and face each other. Sites 8, 9, and 10 are grouped together at the end of the trail, a hike of about 700 feet from your car. I would pick one of these only if the other two in the group were unoccupied—and the chances of that are pretty good on an average non-holiday weekend.

Once you've selected your site, go to site 22 in the main campground to register with the campground host. You can fill water containers at the spigot by the tent-camping parking lot and use the restrooms and showers at the large, clean shower house just across the road in the main campground. The shower house was built in 1997 but is so well maintained that I first thought it was erected much more recently. Although it's usually closed late December through March, I'm told they'll open it up if needed during the winter.

If you want electricity, or just like the convenience of being able to park at your campsite, the main campground also has some beautiful spots on the lake. As you drive into the campground, the first right is a short spur with sites 21 through 25, the shower house, a playground, and the campground host, from whom you can purchase ice and firewood. Next is an intersection, where you'll find the toilet, a soda machine, and an ice machine. Turn right for sites 1 through 20, or go straight or left for sites 26 through 57. This campground is much busier on the weekends, and you'll be sharing with RVs, but the lakeside sites are attractive and fairly large. Check out any of the sites 7 through 16, 34, 35, or 37.

Friends or family who can't handle too much roughing it can reserve (well in advance!) one of the four cabins. These are located next to the tent parking area and offer the same beautiful lakefront view, plus beds for six, a grill, a table and chairs, heat, air-conditioning, fans, and a refrigerator.

The small Dolan Lake Restaurant on the other side of the lake is popular with locals and offers a decent selection of hearty dinners along with sandwiches, salads, and appetizers. They're big into fried food—catfish, bluegill, shrimp, scallops, quail, and frog legs—and whopping steaks—like the 18-ounce T-bone. And where else in Illinois can you get deep-fried dill

MAP

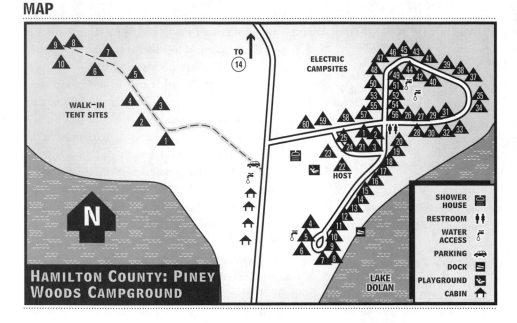

WALK-IN
TENT SITES

TO
(14)

ELECTRIC
CAMPSITES

HOST

SHOWER HOUSE	
RESTROOM	
WATER ACCESS	
PARKING	
DOCK	
PLAYGROUND	
CABIN	

N

HAMILTON COUNTY: PINEY
WOODS CAMPGROUND

LAKE
DOLAN

pickles and cajun-spiced alligator tail? They're open year-round, Thursday to Sunday from 4 to 9 p.m., Sunday for lunch from 11 a.m. to 2 p.m., and for breakfast Saturday and Sunday from 8 a.m. to 11 a.m.

The 75-acre lake was drained in 2006 and refilled and restocked with bass, bluegill, redear, and catfish; crappie will be restocked in the fall of 2008. You can rent rowboats through the restaurant or campground host, but otherwise there's no camp store for purchasing bait, food, or camping supplies. You'll find plenty of stores and restaurants in nearby McLeansboro, though, just 8 miles west on IL 14.

GETTING THERE

From McLeansboro, go
7 miles east on IL 14.
Turn right onto 1625 East
Road at the park sign. Go
1.1 miles south to the park
entrance, on the right.

GPS COORDINATES

UTM Zone 16S
Easting 0376802
Northing 4214138
Latitude N 38° 3' 59.8345"
Longitude W 88° 24' 15.9945"

36
LAKE MURPHYSBORO
STATE PARK

> *Half of the tent sites are as close to the lake as you can get without a boat.*

LOVE CAMPING AT THE WATER'S EDGE, whether it be by a lake, creek, or rolling river. I love it even more when a park like Lake Murphysboro has taken advantage of its miles of shoreline to set up two completely separate lakeside camping areas, one primarily for RVs, and one for tents. And we tent campers get the better deal—our campground is smaller, quieter, and closer to the lake.

As you're coming north off IL 149, turn right toward Lake Murphysboro. If you go straight into the park, you'll come to the popular Big Oak Campground, with 54 electric campsites. Turn left instead, and continue north around the lake 0.5 miles to the two adjacent tent-camping areas (20 sites total). Each site has a table, ground grill, and lantern pole, and most are located on the lakeshore—perfectly situated for fishing, or just sitting and enjoying the view. The first five sites, called Water Lily Campground, are between the main park road and the lake. Site 4 is designated wheelchair-accessible; there are vault toilets directly across the road. Though they're attractive, the primary disadvantage of these sites is their proximity to the road. For that reason, I prefer the sites just around the corner, along the dead-end Shady Rest Campground road.

Shady Rest has 15 sites, half of them as close to the lake as you can get without a boat. Sites 1, 2, and 3 on the right as you enter are good—3 has more space and shade. Sites 4 and 8 are small, but site 5, which is between them, is attractive. All the other sites are spacious, but my favorite is site 15, at the end of the road, which has more room to spread out beneath some tree cover.

Once you've selected a site, register with the campground host at the first site in Big Oak Campground, or settle in and park personnel will come by later. There are vault toilets at both campgrounds, but

RATINGS

Beauty: ✿ ✿ ✿ ✿
Privacy: ✿ ✿ ✿
Spaciousness: ✿ ✿ ✿
Quiet: ✿ ✿ ✿ ✿
Security: ✿ ✿ ✿ ✿
Cleanliness: ✿ ✿ ✿ ✿ ✿

you'll need to get water at the shower house on the other side of the lake.

The tent areas don't fill up as often as the RV campground, but they're still about half full on most good weekends. If you come on a holiday weekend and find it maxed out, the park will open a grassy overflow tent area on the northeast corner of the lake—it's not as pretty, but they'll always find you a spot.

The main park road makes a loop around the lake, a scenic drive with several turnoffs leading to wooded picnic areas on lakeside promontories. On the opposite side of the lake from the campgrounds you'll find the boat launch and shower house, open to all campers from April 1 to mid-November. Lakeside are numerous places to bank fish, as well as a beautiful wooden wheelchair-accessible fishing pier by the docks. There's no longer a concession, but at the park office you can rent johnboats for $10 per day, which includes lifejackets and oars. You can bring your own motor, electric, or gas, 10 horsepower or under.

Considerably more open water and recreational opportunities can be found down the road at nearby Kinkaid Lake. Head straight west out of Lake Murphysboro along Lake Access Road, which becomes Marina Road and curves right at 1.4 miles. Another 1.4 miles brings you to the Kinkaid Village Marina, where you'll find a restaurant, boat rental, groceries, ice, fishing tackle, and bait, as well as a very busy RV campground. This area is hopping on most summer weekends, with hordes of boaters, fishermen, water-skiers, and house-boaters. However, the lake offers 2,750 surface acres, more than 90 miles of shoreline, and almost 9,300 acres of surrounding wilderness, so there are plenty of places to get away from the crowds by boat, foot, or mountain bike.

The lands south and west of Kinkaid Lake are part of the Shawnee National Forest and feature more than 30 miles of fairly rugged trails, with several trailheads and possible routes between them. One beautiful hike begins at the dam at the southern end of the lake and winds north along the lakeshore 3 miles to the Buttermilk Hill picnic area. When you reach the forest service road at the end of the point, turn right to go down to the picnic area and restrooms. (You'll have to retrace

KEY INFORMATION

ADDRESS:	52 Cinder Hill Drive, Murphysboro, IL 62966
OPERATED BY:	IDNR
CONTACT:	(618) 684-2867, www.dnr.state.il.us/lands/landmgt/parks/r5/murphysb.htm
OPEN:	Year-round
SITES:	Class B: 20 nonelectric; Class A: 54 electric
EACH SITE:	Picnic table, fire ring or ground grill, lantern pole
ASSIGNMENT:	First come, first served
REGISTRATION:	Set up and register with host in Big Oak Campground or park staff will come by
FACILITIES:	Water spigots, vault toilets, shower house
PARKING:	At site
FEE:	Class A: $20 per night, $30 per night holidays; Class B: $10 per night
ELEVATION:	494 feet
RESTRICTIONS:	*Pets:* On leash only *Fires:* In fire rings only *Alcohol:* Permitted *Vehicles:* 2 per site *Other:* 14-day limit; 1 RV and 1 tent, or 2 tents per site; 4 adults or 1 family per site

MAP

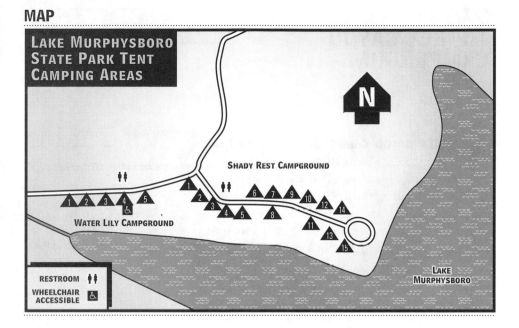

LAKE MURPHYSBORO STATE PARK TENT CAMPING AREAS

SHADY REST CAMPGROUND

WATER LILY CAMPGROUND

RESTROOM
WHEELCHAIR ACCESSIBLE

LAKE MURPHYSBORO

GETTING THERE

From US 51 and IL 13 in Carbondale, go west 7 miles to Murphysboro, where IL 13 becomes IL 149. Continue 3.5 miles west on IL 149 to Lake Access Road, on the right. Turn right and go 0.5 miles to the park entrance, also on the right.

GPS COORDINATES

UTM Zone 16S
Easting 0289623
Northing 4183797
Latitude N 37° 46' 38.3813"
Longitude W 89° 23' 19.6282"

your steps to the dam, since the picnic area is accessible by boat or foot only.) To get to the dam, go west on IL 149 to Spillway Road (just past the bridge). Turn right and head north 1.25 miles to the parking area in front of the gate. The trail begins 0.25 miles up the hill, at the west end of the dam.

For other hiking options around Kinkaid Lake, go to **www.fs.fed.us/r9/forests/shawnee/recreation/rogs** and download the guides to Kinkaid Lake, Gum Ridge, Buttermilk Hill, and Waterfall Trail. (Note that the section between Buttermilk Hill trailhead and the picnic area is temporarily closed.) As on all trails in the Shawnee Forest, be sure to carry water, a map, and a compass or GPS unit.

37
TURKEY BAYOU CAMPGROUND

TURKEY BAYOU CAMPGROUND is located between the Big Muddy River and Turkey Bayou, an abandoned oxbow lake of the Big Muddy. At 338 feet in elevation, this is just about as low as you can go in Illinois. It's surrounded by water and consequently can flood; in fact, from spring to mid-summer you're better off leaving it to the mosquitoes. During the drier, cooler days of fall, however, Turkey Bayou is a great place to camp if you like solitude and don't mind primitive sites. Outside of hunting season, chances are good you'll have the place all to yourself and can use it as a base for exploring some the lesser-known sites of the eastern Shawnee Forest.

> *During the drier, cooler days of fall, Turkey Bayou is a great place to camp in solitude.*

The campground consists of a single loop, with five unnumbered sites, each with a fire ring and table. As you enter, the first site on the right has a gravel base and doesn't offer much shade. The second has more shade but was flooded when I was there in late August. The third and fourth sites are more attractive, being right by the water, but have less shade. The fifth is at the end of the loop, back where it connects with the road in. If flooding is not a concern, I prefer the sites closest to the water. Bring a pole and you can fish right from your campsite. Bring a boat or canoe, and you can explore the river. Don't bring a swimsuit, though—the Big Muddy is aptly named and is home to poisonous cottonmouth snakes.

The U.S. Forest Service keeps Turkey Bayou open for primitive camping but no longer maintains any facilities there—no water, no toilets, and no charge for camping. The area is popular during the hunting seasons, which in southern Illinois span from late November to late January. As you drive past the seasonal wetlands along Oakwood Bottoms Road on the way in, you can understand why this is prime waterfowl-hunting area. To view the wetlands from a dry 0.25-mile boardwalk

RATINGS

Beauty: ✿ ✿ ✿
Privacy: ✿ ✿ ✿ ✿ ✿
Spaciousness: ✿ ✿ ✿
Quiet: ✿ ✿ ✿ ✿ ✿
Security: ✿ ✿ ✿ ✿
Cleanliness: ✿ ✿ ✿ ✿ ✿

ADDRESS:	c/o Mississippi Bluffs Ranger District, 521 North Main Street, Jonesboro, IL 62952
OPERATED BY:	U.S. Forest Service
CONTACT:	(618) 833-8576, www.fs.fed.us/r9/ forests/shawnee/ recreation/ camping/turkey
OPEN:	Year-round
SITES:	5 tent sites
EACH SITE:	Picnic table, fire ring
ASSIGNMENT:	First come, first served
REGISTRATION:	No registration required
FACILITIES:	None
PARKING:	At site
FEE:	Free
ELEVATION:	338 feet
RESTRICTIONS:	*Pets:* On leash only *Fires:* In fire rings only *Alcohol:* Permitted *Vehicles:* 2 per site *Other:* 14-day limit; 8 campers per site

trail, stop at Oakwood Bottoms Greentree Reservoir, 1 mile east of IL 3.

Across the Big Muddy River from the north of the campground you can actually look east into one of the neatest sites to explore in the Shawnee Forest: Little Grand Canyon. To get there, however, you have to get around the Big Muddy and approach from the east. Head 3.5 miles north of Oakwood Bottoms on IL 3 to Town Creek Road, where you'll see a sign for Little Grand Canyon. Turn right, go 5.6 miles to Maple Springs Road, and turn right again (Maple Springs will merge with Hickory Ridge Road). Go 6 miles to Little Grand Canyon Road, turn right, and proceed to the parking area. Three sides of the canyon are made up of steep sandstone bluffs, and its western end opens onto the Big Muddy River. A 3.6-mile loop trail descends into the canyon via steps cut into the rock then climbs back out, offering awesome views of the canyon and the Mississippi valley from the bluff tops. There are two trailheads by the parking lot—I suggest starting at the one by the restrooms and doing the loop clockwise. The sandstone steps are steep and slippery when wet; keep your eyes open for snakes—there are venomous ones around here. Don't descend into the canyon if there is the threat of heavy rain, as it can flood. For a good trail map, visit **www.fs.fed.us/r9/forests/shawnee/ recreation/rogs/little-grand-canyon.pdf.** Note that maps and old trail descriptions mention the Hickory Ridge lookout tower, but all that remains of it are a few concrete blocks by the parking lot.

Between the lowlands of Oakwood Bottoms and the Mississippi River to the west sits Fountain Bluff, a 4-mile-long sandstone hill that rises some 400 feet over the surrounding floodplain. At a distant point in geologic history, the bluff actually overlooked the western shore of the Mississippi River. Glacial ice forced the river westward to its present-day course, leaving Fountain Bluff a virtual island.

Today the hill is virtually unknown to tourists but offers some great views of the Mississippi, secluded canyons, and Native American petroglyphs that have unfortunately been damaged by thoughtless visitors. To get to the bluff, head north on IL 3 from Oakwood Bottoms

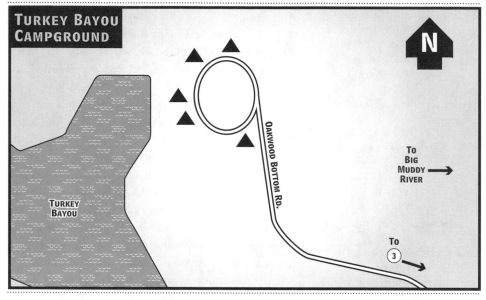

TURKEY BAYOU
CAMPGROUND

N

To
BIG
MUDDY
RIVER

OAKWOOD BOTTOM RD.

TURKEY
BAYOU

To
3

Road. Take the first left onto Happy Hollow Road to drive up the hill and explore from the top. To get to the canyons and petroglyphs, you have to approach from the northwest side. Continue north on IL 3 to Gorham Road, turn left, and go 1.2 miles into town to Second Street. Turn left, and head out of town toward the bluff. At about 1.1 miles, you'll see an isolated grove of trees on the right. Look for a trailhead to the left. Park off to the side; it's a short hike up to the petroglyphs. Just 0.2 miles farther down the road you'll see a parking area on the left. Here you'll find the entrance to a climbable little waterfall canyon leading to three small sandstone shelters. When I was there, someone had erected a couple of makeshift ladders to facilitate access, but one was starting to come apart, so use them with caution.

GETTING THERE

From Murphysboro, head west on IL 149 about 7 miles to IL 3. Turn left and head 5.9 miles south to Oakwood Bottoms Road. Turn left and go 4.5 miles to the campground. From Jonesboro, head west about 8 miles on IL 146 to IL 3. Turn right and drive 17 miles north to Oakwood Bottoms Road. Turn right and it's 4.5 miles to the campground.

GPS COORDINATES

UTM Zone 16S
Easting 0287444
Northing 4173575
Latitude N 37° 41' 5.1814"
Longitude W 89° 24' 37.8568"

Prepare to be awed by the impressive bluffs of the LaRue–Pine Hills.

IF GEOLOGY WERE THE PRIMARY CRITERION, southwestern Illinois around the Pine Hills would belong to neighboring Missouri rather than to Illinois. These narrow ridges and steep hillsides are more reminiscent of the Ozarks to the west and, in fact, represent the easternmost edge of what geologists call the Ozark Uplift. Fortunately for Illinois, the Mississippi River intervened and carved this area from the plateau by its millennia-long wanderings. The result is a virtual island of spectacular bluffs and amazing biodiversity.

In the midst of this, Pine Hills campground is a simple, quiet retreat. With few amenities and only 13 campsites, it doesn't attract RVs, and it is a perfect base camp for exploring the more than 21,000 acres of eastern Shawnee Forest wilderness that surround it.

The campground consists of a single 0.25-mile road, along which the campsites sit. There is no water, but there are vault toilets between sites 10 and 11. Each site has a table, a fire ring, and a lantern post. As you enter the campground, you'll see the signboard and self-registration post on the right. Once you've selected your site, come back here to register and deposit your fee.

Sites 1 through 8 are immediately visible in the first section of the campground, in a grassy clearing with some shade, surrounded by woods. Although sufficiently spacious and spread out, they don't offer much of a sense of privacy. I suggest heading back to sites 9 through 13, which are more separated from the rest of the campground. These offer much better shade and more seclusion. Site 13, at the end of the loop, is my favorite, tucked back into the surrounding woods a bit.

In the past, Pine Hills has been fairly popular—50 to 75 percent full on good weekends. During much of 2008, however, it was closed because a mudslide blocked the road. Usage was down right after it reopened but will probably return to normal in 2009.

RATINGS

Beauty: ☆ ☆ ☆ ☆
Privacy: ☆ ☆ ☆
Spaciousness: ☆ ☆ ☆
Quiet: ☆ ☆ ☆ ☆ ☆
Security: ☆ ☆ ☆ ☆
Cleanliness: ☆ ☆ ☆ ☆ ☆

While at Pine Hills, don't miss the nearby LaRue–Pine Hills Research Natural Area. Here the limestone bluffs of the Ozark plateau face west, overlooking the swamps at their base. You can get there by heading north from the campground on Pine Hills Road, but to appreciate the bluffs you should approach from the west. Take Pine Hills Road south to State Forest Road, then head right to reach IL 3. Turn right again, continue 4.6 miles, and make another right, onto Muddy Levee Road, just before the bridge over Big Muddy River. Follow the Big Muddy for about 2 miles, and then, when you curve to the right, away from the river, the bluffs jump into view. Another 0.5 miles takes you to the base of the bluffs and the intersection with LaRue Road.

From the road below, you may just be able to make out little people looking down from several hundred feet above you. To get to where they are, turn left at the T-intersection, go 0.3 miles, and turn right, onto Pine Hills Road. Go 0.7 miles uphill, to the parking area on the right labeled "Inspiration Point." A 0.25-mile hike will reward you with a panoramic view of the Mississippi River valley below. If you look carefully, you should be able to discern in the swamp the rounded edges of the Mississippi's erstwhile channel. Don't stop there, though. Continue another 500 feet to a couple of other excellent vistas. If you're surefooted and choose to ignore the signs telling you to stay on the trail, there are some obviously worn paths leading out to the bluff's edge.

If you're not herpetophobic, twice a year you can experience another natural wonder at LaRue–Pine Hills, this one biological—the biannual snake migration. The swamp is home to more than half the reptile and amphibian species found in Illinois, including 35 types of snakes. Each fall, with the drop in temperature, they all migrate from the swamp, across LaRue Road to hibernate in the bluffs—then they head back in the spring. A 2.5-mile segment of the road is closed from March 15 to May 15, and from September 1 to October 30 to allow them to cross. You can park at the lot by Winters Pond, just to the right (south) of the junction of Big Muddy Levee Road and LaRue Road, and hike from there. You won't see masses of snakes—on a good day a careful observer may encounter 10 to 20 reptiles along the 2.5 miles.

KEY INFORMATION

ADDRESS:	c/o Mississippi Bluffs Ranger District, 521 North Main Street, Jonesboro, IL 62952
OPERATED BY:	U.S. Forest Service
CONTACT:	(618) 833-8576, www.fs.fed.us/r9/forests/shawnee/recreation/camping/pinehills
OPEN:	Mar. 16–Dec. 14
SITES:	13 tent sites
EACH SITE:	Picnic table, fire ring, lantern pole
ASSIGNMENT:	First come, first served
REGISTRATION:	Self-registration post at entrance
FACILITIES:	Vault toilets
PARKING:	At site
FEE:	$10 per night
ELEVATION:	415 feet
RESTRICTIONS:	*Pets:* On leash only *Fires:* In fire rings only *Alcohol:* Permitted *Vehicles:* 2 per site *Other:* 14-day limit; 8 campers per site

MAP

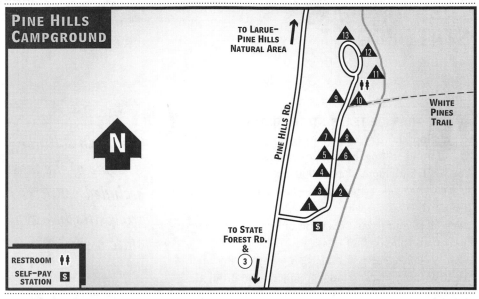

PINE HILLS CAMPGROUND

TO LARUE–PINE HILLS NATURAL AREA

PINE HILLS RD.

WHITE PINES TRAIL

TO STATE FOREST RD. & ③

RESTROOM

SELF–PAY STATION

GETTING THERE

From Jonesboro, take IL 146 west to IL 3. Turn right, go 4.25 miles north to State Forest Road. Turn right again and go 0.6 miles east to Pine Hills Road. Turn left and drive 0.7 miles north to the campground entrance, on the right.

From Murphysboro, take IL 127 south 21 miles to State Forest Road. Turn right and go 7 miles west to Pine Hills Road. Turn right again and proceed as above.

GPS COORDINATES

UTM Zone 16S
Easting 0285849
Northing 4154709
Latitude N 37° 30' 52.2130"
Longitude W 89° 25' 23.0746"

Hikers can explore many miles of rugged trails in the area, starting with White Pine Trail, which begins just behind campsite 10. The trail comes to a junction at about 0.8 miles—continuing straight ahead another 1.2 miles takes you to the clear waters of Hutchins Creek, while heading left takes you along the ridgeline another 2.2 miles to Allen's Flat picnic area on Pine Hills Road. A good trail description can be found at **www.illinois .sierraclub.org/shawnee/unclebob/whitepines.htm;** visit **www.fs.fed.us/r9/forests/shawnee/recreation/rogs/white-pine-trail.pdf** for a map. If you're more ambitious, try the 6-mile Godwin Trail, which crosses the Clear Springs and Bald Knob Wilderness areas. The western trailhead is on Pine Hills Road, about 5.7 miles north of the campground. A trail map can be found at **www.fs.fed.us/ r9/forests/shawnee/recreation/rogs/sh-godwin-trail-rog-2006.pdf.** For this and other wilderness trails, a topographic map and compass or GPS unit are highly recommended.

39
TRAIL OF TEARS
STATE FOREST

AT TRAIL OF TEARS STATE FOREST you won't find showers, electricity, playgrounds, swimming, fishing, boating, or even a pop machine. You will find more than 5,000 acres of beautiful, densely wooded, rugged hills—the easternmost outliers of the Ozarks, with the long, narrow ridges and steep slopes more characteristic of neighboring Missouri than Illinois. Best of all, you will find 14 of the most secluded yet accessible campsites at any state park, where you can camp in solitude far from the nearest neighbor—assuming anyone else is even camping there.

Enter Trail of Tears on State Forest Road, which runs along an east–west valley. From there, two half-loop single-lane gravel roads climb into the hills to the north and south, follow a ridgetop, and descend again. Along each is sprinkled a handful of campsites, most of them excellent. Each has one or two tables, a ground grill, and a trashcan, and most have a pit toilet right at the site. (It may be an outhouse, but at least it's your own private outhouse!) I especially like the sturdy three-sided wooden Adirondack shelters found at four sites, built in the 1930s by the Civilian Conservation Corps. Each has a fireplace, and you can even camp in the shelter—pitch your tent on the floor, or simply hang a tarp over the entrance.

North Forest Road is 4.2 miles long; follow it one-way counterclockwise, starting from its eastern junction with State Forest Road. Head uphill, and you'll first see site N1 (on the left), and then N2 (600 feet farther down the road), with a vault toilet between them. Another 0.25 miles brings you to N4 (on the left), then 1,000 feet later to N5; there's a toilet between these as well. All these sites are spacious and well shaded, but N2 is the largest and most attractive, perched on a ridge over a narrow wooded valley. Two adjacent sites, Y1 and Y2,

> *Camp in solitude at some of the most secluded yet accessible campsites in any state park.*

RATINGS

Beauty: ✰ ✰ ✰ ✰
Privacy: ✰ ✰ ✰ ✰ ✰
Spaciousness: ✰ ✰ ✰ ✰ ✰
Quiet: ✰ ✰ ✰ ✰ ✰
Security: ✰ ✰ ✰ ✰
Cleanliness: ✰ ✰ ✰ ✰ ✰

KEY INFORMATION

ADDRESS:	3240 State Forest Road, Jonesboro IL 62952
OPERATED BY:	IDNR
CONTACT:	(618) 833-4910, www.dnr.state.il.us/lands/land mgt/parks/r5/trltears.htm
OPEN:	Year-round (hike-in only season Dec. 24–mid-May; all sites become hike-in during that period, when roads are closed)
SITES:	Class C: 14; multiple hike-in sites; 1 group site
EACH SITE:	Table, ground grill, trashcan; 4 sites have 3-sided wooden shelter
ASSIGNMENT:	Reservations accepted in person or by mail only; otherwise, first come, first served
REGISTRATION:	Set up and park staff will come by
FACILITIES:	Water spigot, vault toilets
PARKING:	At campsite; along road (hike-in sites)
FEE:	Class C: $8 per tent per night; hike-in sites: $6 per tent per night
ELEVATION:	472 feet
RESTRICTIONS:	*Pets:* On leash only *Fires:* In fire rings only *Alcohol:* Permitted *Vehicles:* 2 per site

are located at the northernmost point of the road. From here the road starts downhill, passing N6, N7, and N8, on the right, and finally N9, on the left at the bottom of the hill. N6 and N8 are beautiful—each has one of the large shelters, plenty of grassy space, and shade. N7 doesn't have a shelter and is a bit smaller, but it's still a great site. N9 is located in a large open clearing amid woods and doesn't have the view or shade of the sites farther uphill.

The other four campsites are along the 2.5 miles of South Forest Road, which also runs one-way, counterclockwise, beginning just across from the white barn housing the visitor center. Cross the concrete ford through the stream, head past the picnic area on the left, and climb the hill. From the T-intersection at the top of the hill, site S1 is on the right. You'll find one of the wooden shelters here, but it's smaller than the others, and the area in front of it is gravel. For a better option, turn left at the T-intersection and go 1.3 miles to site S2, my favorite spot on the south side; it has a larger shelter and plenty of space for multiple tents. Farther down the road are sites S3 and S4. Neither has a wooden shelter, but both are good—well shaded and spacious.

Youth or adult groups can camp by prior arrangement at the group area, which is off the south road. This area features a large shelter, a grill, a big fire ring surrounded by benches, and a neat outdoor amphitheater.

Wherever you settle, you'll need to get water at the spigot in front of the white barn. If park personnel are there, you can register, or just set up camp and they'll come around later. Note that, unlike at most other state parks, fees here are per tent, not per site. You can reserve a site in advance by mail or in person for an additional $5—a good idea if you want a particular shelter. Reservations are necessary only during hunting season, just before and after Thanksgiving. Camping is permitted year-round, but the north and south roads are closed from December 24 through mid-May, so it's hike-in only then.

You can also backpack camp almost anywhere in the forest that's away from established campsites or picnic areas. Obtain a permit first from the visitor center

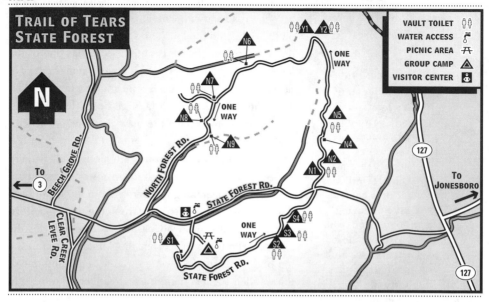

(or check at the maintenance building behind the center) and be sure your vehicle doesn't block a road or fire lane.

Trail of Tears offers miles of hiking, equestrian, and fire trails, much of it fairly strenuous due to the hilly terrain. Be sure to bring a trail map (from the park brochure or Web site) and a compass or GPS unit because the trails are complex. A moderately difficult and pretty 2-mile trail loops through the Ozark Hills Nature Preserve on the south side. The trailhead is located between campsites S3 and S4.

While at Trail of Tears, don't miss the Pomona Natural Bridge, just 15 miles north. You can cross over and under this impressive 90-foot sandstone arch via a 0.3-mile loop trail. Take IL 127 north 10.8 miles to Pomona Road and turn left. Go 0.8 miles west to the three-way stop, turn right, and proceed 2.3 miles to the parking area.

Check the profiles of nearby Pine Hills and Turkey Bayou campgrounds for many other sites to explore in the eastern Shawnee National Forest.

GETTING THERE

From US 51 and IL 146 at Anna, go 5 miles west on IL 146 to IL 127. Turn right and go 1.25 miles north to State Forest Road on the left. Turn left and drive 1.25 miles to the forest entrance.

GPS COORDINATES

UTM Zone 16S
Easting 0293839
Northing 4151582
Latitude North 37° 29' 17.3778"
Longitude West 89° 19' 54.7113"

> *Do not miss the chance to hike amid the fascinating rock formations that have earned this park its name.*

GIANT CITY STATE PARK has something for everyone. Whether you enjoy rappelling, horseback riding, or relaxing in the air-conditioned comfort of a completely furnished cabin, you'll find it here. A prime attraction is the hiking: trek amid the fascinating rock formations that have earned this park its name. Tent campers have their own separate area, and though it can seem crowded on busy weekends, it's well worth it to experience all this beautiful park has to offer.

If you enter the park from the north on Giant City Road, turn left onto the first road, toward the campground. If entering from Makanda or US 51, take the first left and then the second right onto the campground road. Turn right into the campground, where you'll find the host's site on the right. If the host is in, you can register there; otherwise, set up camp and park personnel will come by later.

The 85 Class A electric sites in the main campground are average RV sites. To find a better choice for tent camping, go all the way to the south end of the campground on the middle road to reach the parking area for the walk-in tent-camping sites. There are 14 campsites here—each with a table and ground grill—scattered around a grassy area that is shaded by pine and deciduous trees. These are farther apart than the RV sites, but there still isn't much brush between them—you and your neighbors will have to pretend you have more privacy than you really do.

And almost any time during the regular camping season you will have neighbors. Giant City is popular, and even the tent sites can fill on fair-weather weekends. For that reason I suggest walking the 200-feet or so to one of the sites farthest from the road—4, 5, 7, 8, or 9. You'll be out of the flow of traffic to the other sites, will have a bit more shade, and still won't feel as

RATINGS

Beauty: ☆ ☆ ☆
Privacy: ☆ ☆
Spaciousness: ☆ ☆ ☆
Quiet: ☆ ☆ ☆
Security: ☆ ☆ ☆ ☆ ☆
Cleanliness: ☆ ☆ ☆ ☆ ☆

crowded as you would in the RV campground—but you can use the same modern shower house.

Backpackers can try the 12-mile Red Cedar Trail, which has eight primitive sites with toilets (but no water) at the 6-mile point on the trail. Register first with the campground host or park office, and park at the trailhead by the walk-in sites. Even here, though, you may not find seclusion on the weekends, since these sites are popular with students from nearby Southern Illinois University.

Do not miss the chance to hike at Giant City. To best appreciate what you'll see, first stop at the visitor center to view the displays and a short film about the geology of the area and pick up the detailed hiking guides for each trail. Kids can explore hands-on exhibits in the Discovery Corner. Then take the 1-mile Giant City Trail, which winds through sandstone blocks left after eons of erosion created what today seem like "avenues" amid the buildings of a city for giants—hence the park's name. Kids love to scramble around these. Other short trails lead past sandstone bluffs, inspiring overlooks, a cool shelter cave, and the remnants of a stone wall left by Native Americans.

Even if you enjoy roughing it, spend a few minutes indoors at the rustic and comfortable Giant City Lodge. This building was constructed by the Civilian Conservation Corps in the 1930s from local sandstone and white-oak timbers and has been renovated and expanded, maintaining its historic beauty. To get away from campfire cooking, try their excellent Bald Knob dining room before you leave, taking advantage of the all-you-can-eat family-style fried chicken dinner, served on Sundays from 11:30 a.m. to 4 p.m. Friends or family who'd rather have a bed can rent one of the fully furnished cabins and swim in the pool during the summer. Check **www.giant citylodge.com** or call (618) 457-4921 for reservations.

Horseback riding for kids and adults is available through Giant City Stables, a private concession in the park. They offer guided trail rides of one to three hours, lessons, and pony rides for the younger wranglers. You can get more information and current rates at (618) 529-4110 or **www.giantcitystables.com.**

Rock climbing and rappelling are permitted in two places—at the bluffs by Devil's Standtable and at

ADDRESS:	235 Giant City Rd., Makanda, IL
OPERATED BY:	IDNR
CONTACT:	(618) 457-4836, www.dnr.state.il. us/lands/landmgt/ parks/r5/gc.htm
OPEN:	Year-round
SITES:	Class C: 14 walk-in sites; Class A: 85 sites
EACH SITE:	Picnic table, fire ring; electric (Class A only)
ASSIGNMENT:	First come, first served
REGISTRATION:	Register with campground host (if available) or set up and park staff will come by
FACILITIES:	Water spigots, vault toilets, shower house (closed Jan.–Feb.)
PARKING:	Class A: at site; Class C and backpacking: in lot
FEE:	Class A: $20 per night, $30 per night holidays; Class C and backpacking: $8 per night
ELEVATION:	676 feet
RESTRICTIONS:	*Pets:* On leash only *Fires:* In fire rings only *Alcohol:* Permitted in campground only *Vehicles:* 2 per site *Other:* 14-day limit; 1 RV and 1 tent, or 2 tents per site; 4 adults or 1 family per site

MAP

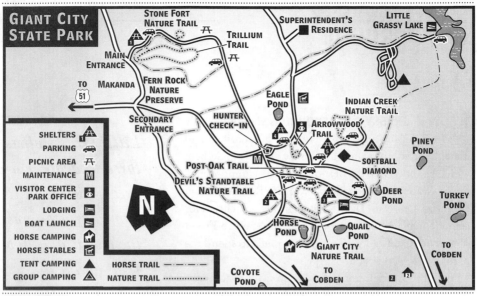

GIANT CITY STATE PARK

STONE FORT NATURE TRAIL
SUPERINTENDENT'S RESIDENCE
LITTLE GRASSY LAKE
TRILLIUM TRAIL
MAIN ENTRANCE
TO MAKANDA
US 51
FERN ROCK NATURE PRESERVE
SECONDARY ENTRANCE
HUNTER CHECK-IN
EAGLE POND
INDIAN CREEK NATURE TRAIL
ARROWWOOD TRAIL
PINEY POND
POST-OAK TRAIL
DEVIL'S STANDTABLE NATURE TRAIL
SOFTBALL DIAMOND
DEER POND
TURKEY POND
HORSE POND
QUAIL POND
GIANT CITY NATURE TRAIL
TO COBDEN
COYOTE POND
TO COBDEN

SHELTERS
PARKING
PICNIC AREA
MAINTENANCE
VISITOR CENTER PARK OFFICE
LODGING
BOAT LAUNCH
HORSE CAMPING
HORSE STABLES
TENT CAMPING
GROUP CAMPING

HORSE TRAIL ---------
NATURE TRAIL ·············

GETTING THERE

From the north, take I-57 to IL 13 West (Exit 54B). Drive west 13 miles to Giant City Road (there's a light, and a Wal-Mart on the right). Turn left and go 12 miles south.

From the south, take I-57 to IL 148 West (Exit 45). Go 3 miles northwest to Grassy Road. Turn left. Go 9 miles to T-intersection with Giant City Road (stay left at fork at about 4.5 miles). Turn left and drive 4 miles to the park.

GPS COORDINATES

UTM Zone 16S
Easting 0307311
Northing 4164837
Latitude N 37° 36' 37.6596"
Longitude W 89° 10' 59.0535"

Shelter #1. No check-in or registration is necessary—just be sure you know what you're doing, bring your own equipment, and understand that you climb at your own risk. No permanent anchors are allowed, and remember that wet sandstone can be slippery.

If you want another hike amid interesting geology, head for Rocky Bluff Trail at nearby Devil's Kitchen Lake. From Giant City, go 3 miles north on Giant City Road to Little Grassy Road and turn right. Drive 3.5 miles to Tacoma Lake Road, turn right, and go 0.5 miles to the Rocky Bluff trailhead parking. This 1.8-mile loop will take you past seasonal waterfalls and sandstone cliffs. Devil's Kitchen Lake is part of the Crab Orchard National Wildlife Refuge, so a $2-per-day vehicle tag is necessary and can be purchased at one of the refuge campgrounds.

LITTLE GRASSY CAMPGROUND

LITTLE GRASSY CAMPGROUND is serendipitously included in this book—I almost missed it. I had intended to camp at nearby Devil's Kitchen, which sounded like the best of the three campgrounds in the Crab Orchard National Wildlife Refuge for tent camping. However, Devil's Kitchen was still closed for remodeling—I could visit, but I couldn't stay. So I went down the road to Little Grassy for a place to spend the night and was pleasantly surprised.

Little Grassy Campground is on a 1,200-acre lake of the same name and is operated as a private concession under the U.S. Fish & Wildlife Service, which manages the almost 44,000 acres of the entire wildlife refuge. It has three RV camping areas, which were full when I visited, and struck me as claustrophobically tight. However, Little Grassy also offers three separate tent-only areas, each with its own character and all virtually empty. Even on a busy weekend, rarely more than half the tent sites are occupied, so you should be able to find a quiet spot.

As you drive into the campground, take the first right to Sam's Point, one of the three tent areas. Fourteen sites are situated along the road that extends to the tip of the point and the lakeshore. Campsites here are open and grassy, with some shade, and a few choice spots are right by the water's edge. Site 1, off to the right as you enter, is the largest and is well away from the road. Sites 7, 8, and 9, at the end of the point, are my favorites. Only sites 4 and 5 were too small, in my estimation.

Past the Sam's Point entrance, you'll see a cluster of RVs on the right. Turn left instead to take the road angling back into the Woodview tent area. As the name suggests, these 11 sites, though not as spacious, have plenty of tree cover. If possible, head for the end of the point—site 21 is beautiful, the most secluded in the

> *Little Grassy offers three separate tent-only areas, each with its own character, one in the woods and two right on the lake.*

RATINGS

Beauty: ✿ ✿ ✿
Privacy: ✿ ✿ ✿
Spaciousness: ✿ ✿ ✿
Quiet: ✿ ✿ ✿ ✿
Security: ✿ ✿ ✿ ✿ ✿
Cleanliness: ✿ ✿ ✿ ✿

ADDRESS:	788 Hidden Bay Lane, Makanda, IL 62958
OPERATED BY:	Private concession, under Crab Orchard National Wildlife Refuge, U.S. Fish & Wildlife Service
CONTACT:	(618) 457-6655
OPEN:	Apr. 1–Oct. 31
SITES:	37 tent sites, 66 electric and water sites, 12 full hookup sites
EACH SITE:	Picnic table, ground grill
ASSIGNMENT:	First come, first served
REGISTRATION:	Register at the marina office
FACILITIES:	Water spigot, shower house with flush toilets, beach
PARKING:	At site
FEE:	$13 per night tent sites, $17 per night electric and water sites, $24 per night full-hookup sites
ELEVATION:	566 feet
RESTRICTIONS:	*Pets:* On leash only *Fires:* In fire rings only *Alcohol:* Not permitted *Vehicles:* 2 per site *Other:* 1 RV and 1 tent; 6 people per site

entire campground, and overlooks the lake below. Site 22 is almost as nice, with a similar view, and sites 20 and 23 are also good.

Opposite the Woodview entrance, the low road to the right leads to Tenter's Hill, where 12 sites perch on a hillside that slopes gradually down the lakeshore. These sites don't have the shade of Woodview but are ideal if you like camping by the water's edge. Sites 26 and 27 are fairly spacious and a bit more secluded. Sites 28 and 31 have the best lake view. Sites 32 through 35 on the shore are too close to one another, but any one would be great if the others weren't occupied. I'd avoid sites 36 and 37, which are virtually in the backyard of the RV section above.

Once you've selected your site, go to the marina at the end of the campground road to register. You can purchase snacks and drinks at the small store there. If you're going to explore any other sites in the wildlife refuge (see the chapter on Devil's Kitchen for possibilities), you'll need a vehicle pass, which can be purchased here as well.

The main inconvenience at Little Grassy is that the only restrooms are in the shower house, located along the main road past the entrance to Woodview. Depending on the campsite, you may have to walk as far as 0.1 mile—not a long hike, but not fun in the middle of the night. Less critical, the only public water spigot is at the entrance to Sam's Point.

From Memorial Day weekend to Labor Day, the campground beach is open from 7 a.m. to 7 p.m., with a lifeguard on duty from 11 a.m. Don't imagine diving or swimming laps, however—the beach is small, and the water only 4 feet deep at most. Let the kids splash around while you sit in the water and cool off.

Boat fishing is a popular pastime on Little Grassy Lake, and the tree-lined shores are worth exploring in their own right. You can rent motorboats at the marina. If you bring your own motor, note that there's a 10-horsepower limit. You'll need to purchase a refuge boat pass from the marina as well.

Young anglers in particular may enjoy visiting the Little Grassy Fish Hatchery, 0.5 miles north of the campground on Grassy Road. This Illinois Department

MAP

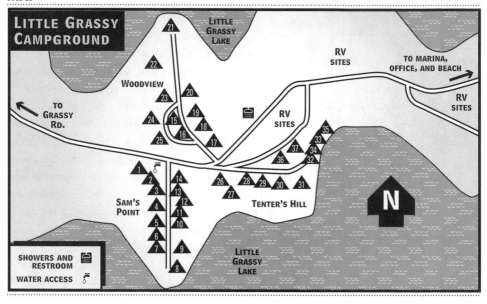

LITTLE GRASSY CAMPGROUND

LITTLE GRASSY LAKE

RV SITES

TO MARINA, OFFICE, AND BEACH

RV SITES

WOODVIEW

TO GRASSY RD.

RV SITES

SAM'S POINT

TENTER'S HILL

N

LITTLE GRASSY LAKE

SHOWERS AND RESTROOM

WATER ACCESS

---

of Natural Resources' facility produces 15 million fish annually, including channel catfish, largemouth bass, redear, bluegill, walleye, and muskie. The hatchery is open for free tours every day from 8:00 a.m. to 3:30 p.m., though from November to February there are no fish to see. During July and August visitors can feed the catfish in the outdoor raceways. For more details, check **www.dnr.state.il.us/lands/education/interprt/litgras.htm** or call (618) 529-4100.

Little Grassy Campground is also a good base from which to explore nearby (and typically much busier) Giant City State Park. Hike among the amazing geological formations, have dinner at the historic lodge, and return at night to your quiet campsite on the shores of Little Grassy Lake.

GPS COORDINATES

UTM Zone 16S
Easting 0310261
Northing 4168381
Latitude N 37° 38' 34.7897"
Longitude W 89° 9' 2.1118"

GETTING THERE

From I-57, take Exit 45 to IL 148 and head northwest 2.8 miles to Grassy Road. Turn left and follow Grassy Road 11 miles to Hidden Bay Lane, on the left (watch for the "Camp Carew" sign). Make a left and it's less than 0.5 miles to the campground. From IL 13 and US 51 in Carbondale, go 1.9 miles east to Giant City Road. Turn right and go 6.75 miles south to Grassy Road. Turn left and drive 0.5 miles to Hidden Bay Lane, on the right. Turn right and it's less than 0.5 miles to the campground.

> *Unique to Devil's Kitchen Campground are the individual boat slips, one for each campsite.*

THE CAMPGROUND AT DEVIL'S KITCHEN LAKE has been around for a while—but it is also brand-new. It was formerly a 45-site RV campground privately operated under license from the U.S. Fish & Wildlife Service, which owns the almost 44,000 acres of Crab Orchard National Wildlife Refuge in which the campground is located. In 2006, however, Fish & Wildlife decided to assume direct management and return the area to a more primitive state, allowing only tent camping. It was closed in 2007 and 2008 for remodeling and will reopen in the spring of 2009 as a small, quiet campground surrounded by rocky out-croppings on a scenic, tree-lined lake.

The signboard at the entrance to Devil's Kitchen Campground is where you self-register after selecting your site. To use any of the facilities within the refuge (lakes, boat ramps, parking areas, or trails), you also need a vehicle pass, which you can purchase here.

The wood-encircled camping area is on a large grass-covered point that juts into the northern end of Devil's Kitchen Lake. Eight primitive walk-in sites form a circle around the clearing and cedar posts and railings border each site, which has its own table, ground grill, and lantern post. The closest disabled-accessible site is by the parking lot; the farthest is about 250 feet away. The sites are fairly far apart and have some shade, though there's not much brush separating them. If all eight were occupied, it might feel busy, but with so few sites, this should still be a quiet spot. You'll find a water spigot in the middle of the campground, and the shower house and restrooms are just across the parking lot.

Wildlife is abundant around Devil's Kitchen. You may see a beaver swimming by in the evening, deer by the restrooms, or a family of raccoons near the campground. The refuge as a whole is home to more than 260 bird species, including some nesting pairs of bald eagles.

RATINGS

Beauty: ✪ ✪ ✪ ✪
Privacy: ✪ ✪ ✪
Spaciousness: ✪ ✪ ✪
Quiet: ✪ ✪ ✪ ✪
Security: ✪ ✪ ✪ ✪ ✪
Cleanliness: ✪ ✪ ✪ ✪ ✪

Unique to Devil's Kitchen Campground are the individual boat docks, one for each campsite. Take the short trail down from the parking area to the little inlet, where you'll find eight beautiful wooden boat slips. The campground is primitive, but the boat slips have lights and electrical hookups. The boat ramp is down the road just before the campground entrance. Note that boats using the lake must have a pass, available from the refuge visitor center on IL 148 in Carbondale or from the marina at Little Grassy Lake. Boats on Devil's Kitchen must be 10 horsepower or less.

It's hard to say how popular the campground will be when it reopens in 2009, since it has been closed for two years. With various other camping options nearby (Giant City, Little Grassy, Crab Orchard), I'm hoping Devil's Kitchen stays relatively unnoticed for a while.

All three of the refuge lakes are popular for boating and fishing. Crab Orchard is the largest lake, at 6,900 acres, and is busy with sailboats and water-skiers on warm summer days. Crappie and largemouth bass fishing are excellent. On the northwest end, just off Spillway Road, south of IL 13, there's a full-service marina where you can rent boats. The 1,200-acre Little Grassy Lake, to the west of Devil's Kitchen, is quieter and also has a marina and a small beach. Devil's Kitchen covers 810 acres and has been intentionally left the least developed. With a maximum depth of 90 feet, it is also the second-deepest lake in Illinois (surpassed only by Lake Michigan), and the crystal-clear, cool waters are ideal for rainbow trout. This is one of the few places in southern Illinois where you can fish for trout year-round. For more details and a map of all the refuge lakes and ponds, pick up the Crab Orchard fishing brochure at the campground signboard.

Three of the refuge's five established hiking trails are located around Devil's Kitchen Lake. If you have time for just one, take the 1.8-mile Rocky Bluff loop trail. The trailhead is about 0.5 miles south of the campground, on Tacoma Lake Road (there is parking on the left). This moderately difficult loop will take you through sandstone canyons and past seasonal waterfalls and shelter caves. It is especially beautiful (and popular) in the spring, when wildflowers of all colors carpet the

KEY INFORMATION

ADDRESS: Tacoma Lake Road, Makanda, IL, 62958; Crab Orchard office: 8588 Route 148, Marion, IL 62959

OPERATED BY: Crab Orchard National Wildlife Refuge, U.S. Fish & Wildlife Service

CONTACT: Crab Orchard office: (618) 997-3344, www.fws.gov/midwest/craborchard (no specific campground Web site)

OPEN: Apr. 1–Oct. 31

SITES: 8 walk-in tent sites

EACH SITE: Picnic table, fire ring, lantern post

ASSIGNMENT: First come, first served

REGISTRATION: Self-registration

FACILITIES: Water spigot, shower house with flush toilets, boat slips

PARKING: In lot

FEE: $10 per night

ELEVATION: 545 feet

RESTRICTIONS: *Pets:* On leash only
Fires: In fire rings only
Alcohol: Not permitted
Vehicles: 2 per site
Other: 14-day limit; 8 people per site

MAP

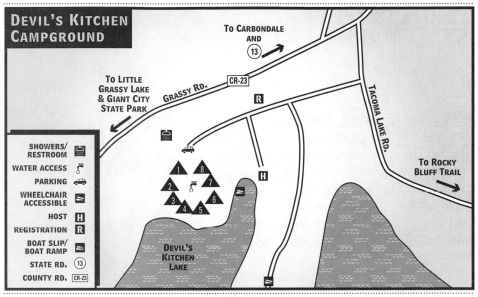

DEVIL'S KITCHEN CAMPGROUND

TO CARBONDALE AND (13)

TO LITTLE GRASSY LAKE & GIANT CITY STATE PARK

GRASSY RD.   CR-23

TACOMA LAKE RD.

TO ROCKY BLUFF TRAIL

SHOWERS/RESTROOM
WATER ACCESS
PARKING
WHEELCHAIR ACCESSIBLE
HOST **H**
REGISTRATION **R**
BOAT SLIP/BOAT RAMP
STATE RD. (13)
COUNTY RD. CR-23

DEVIL'S KITCHEN LAKE

GETTING THERE

From I-57, take Exit 54 in Marion, go west 10.2 miles on IL 13, and make the first left after crossing Crab Orchard Lake onto Spillway Road. Follow Spillway Road 9 miles (it joins Grassy Road at 8 miles) to Tacoma Lake Road. Turn left, then make the first right into the campground. From US 51 and IL 13 in Carbondale, go 4.1 miles east to Spillway Road, turn right, go 9 miles south, and proceed as above at Tacoma Lake Road.

canyon floor. Note that the trail can be muddy and the wet sandstone slippery.

Offering scenic views of Devil's Kitchen Lake, Grassy Creek Trail is a 1.4-mile loop with a wide, paved surface that was once an old road. To get to the trail parking, head south on Tacoma Lake Road about 2.9 miles from the campground, then turn right and drive 0.5 miles just over Grassy Creek Bridge. Maps and descriptions of all the trails are available at the refuge visitor center, where you can pick up a printed guide for the 9-mile auto tour of the refuge as well. You can also take the longer Fall Discovery Auto Tour, which takes you through otherwise closed areas, but this is only available on Sunday afternoons in October.

GPS COORDINATES

UTM Zone 16S
Easting 0314311
Northing 4168686
Latitude N 37° 38' 47.6532"
Longitude W 89° 6' 17.2263"

43

FERNE CLYFFE STATE PARK

BEFORE I EVER CONTEMPLATED writing this book, Ferne Clyffe was my favorite place to camp in Illinois. I'm almost done visiting campgrounds for this book, and it still is. Somehow the combination of beautiful, secluded, comfortable campsites and excellent hiking draws me back again and again. Since it's right in the middle of southern Illinois, it's also a great base from which to explore the Shawnee Forest to the east and west.

Enter the park off IL 37, and go 0.5 miles to the stop sign. Uphill and straight ahead is the RV campground—turn left instead. At the Y-intersection by the lake, you may be sorely tempted to stop (as I am) to simply sit on the bench and take in the tranquil view—save that for later. Take the left fork, and follow the signs to Turkey Ridge tent camping (turn right, then left).

This campground must have been designed by a tent camper. Each of the 20 sites is a short walk from parking, yet most are far enough apart and surrounded by plenty of trees and brush to let you feel like you're all alone. All are beautifully shaded, and many are on raised flat pads bordered by landscaping timbers. Each has a ground grill, table, and lantern post, and all campers can use the main campground's shower building (closed from the Monday before Thanksgiving until April 1).

My favorite site is 10: all the way at the end, it is large, flat, and well secluded from its only neighbor, site 9. Because it's on a hill below the level of the parking lot, you can't even see the lot from the site. Sites 1–9 are tucked away in the woods, accessed by short trails—1 is probably the best of these, as long as there's no one at nearby site 2. Sites 11 and 12 are attractive and spacious but a bit close to parking for me. Sites 13 through 18 are all in the woods, off a short half-circle trail. Watch for poison ivy—it abounds off the trails around sites 1 through 10.

> *Ferne Clyffe is a hiker's paradise.*

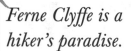

RATINGS

Beauty: ✪ ✪ ✪ ✪ ✪
Privacy: ✪ ✪ ✪ ✪
Spaciousness: ✪ ✪ ✪ ✪ ✪
Quiet: ✪ ✪ ✪ ✪ ✪
Security: ✪ ✪ ✪ ✪
Cleanliness: ✪ ✪ ✪ ✪ ✪

ADDRESS: Route 37, P.O. Box 10, Goreville, IL

OPERATED BY: IDNR

CONTACT: (618) 995-2411, www.dnr.state.il.us/lands/landmgt/parks/r5/ferne.htm

OPEN: Year-round (backpacking sites closed third weekend in Nov. to first weekend in Dec.)

SITES: Class B: 20 walk-in (Turkey Ridge), Class A: 59 sites (Deer Ridge)

EACH SITE: Picnic table, fire ring; electric (Class A only)

ASSIGNMENT: First come, first served

REGISTRATION: Register with host in Deer Ridge or set up and park staff will come by

FACILITIES: Flush toilets, showers (Deer Ridge, available to all), water spigots, vault toilets

PARKING: At site (Deer Ridge); in lot (Turkey Ridge and backpacking sites)

FEE: Deer Ridge: $20 per night, $30 per night on holidays; all others: $8 per night

ELEVATION: 712 feet

RESTRICTIONS: *Pets:* On leash only
Fires: In fire rings only
Alcohol: Permitted
Vehicles: 2 per site
Other: 14-day limit; 1 RV and 1 tent, or 2 tents per site; 4 adults or 1 family per site

If Turkey Ridge is full (possible on spring or fall weekends), or if you'd like more privacy, there are three backpacking sites. Take the backpack trail at the end of the parking lot for a 0.75-mile hike downhill and then, unfortunately, back up—a bit of work if you're hauling stuff. There's also a simple shortcut: go between sites 1 and 2, cut across a short bit of woods until you reach an obvious trail, and turn left. You've just bypassed the downhill-uphill part, and now it's only 0.2 level miles to the backpack sites. These sites are in the woods and each has a fire ring and table. You may be surprised to see a road just a little farther on that leads to the rarely occupied equestrian camping area, where you can use the toilets and water spigot.

Ferne Clyffe is a hiker's paradise. There are 18 well-marked hiking trails, ranging from 0.25 to 8 miles in length, which take you along high sandstone bluffs, through cool canyons, and by seasonal waterfalls and shelter bluff caves. Many of the trails connect, and it's helpful to have the map and trail descriptions handy; find them on the park Web site or in the brochure. Many of the most popular trails can be accessed from the parking loop at the end of the picnic shelter road—take the right fork at the Y-intersection by the lake. Some of the "ooh-ahh" sights are actually not too far from here—nice if you have kids who aren't up for a long trek. Hawk's Cave Trail is an easy 0.5-mile loop leading to a 150-foot sandstone cave, and a 100-foot seasonal waterfall is an easy 0.75-mile round-trip via Big Rocky Hollow Trail.

Rock climbing and rappelling are permitted in two areas of the park, off Rebman Trail and at Cedar Bluff. No permission or certification is required—climb at your own risk, and be sure you know what you're doing. And if you don't know what you're doing but would like to learn, check out Vertical Heartland, just 8 miles southwest of Ferne Clyffe. At this privately owned portion of Draper's Bluff, Eric Ulner offers half-day and full-day climbing instruction for individuals, families, and groups—no experience is required. Call (618) 995-1427 for a reservation, or check **www.verticalheartland.com** for more information.

South of Ferne Clyffe is the unique Cache River State Natural Area, almost 15,000 acres of wetlands that

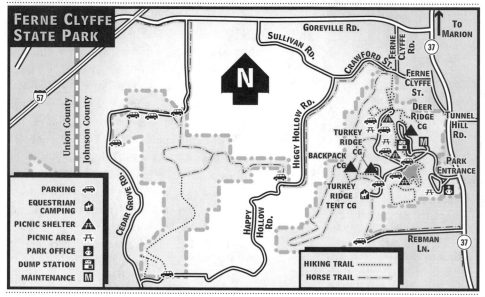

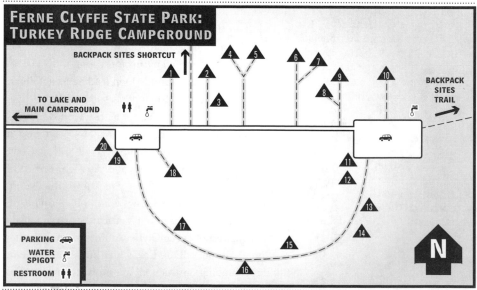

look like the Louisiana bayou. You can explore various trails and boardwalks over the swamp—don't miss the state's oldest living resident, a bald cypress tree that's more than 1,000 years old and has a base circumference of more than 40 feet. Start at the excellent Barkhausen Wetlands Visitor Center, 16.5 miles south of the Ferne Clyffe entrance on IL 37, open Wednesday through Sunday, 9 a.m. to 4 p.m. Call (618) 657-2064 for information. There is also a fascinating, well-marked canoe trail through the lower Cache River. Unfortunately, as of 2008 there was no canoe outfitter serving the Cache.

Cyclists may want to try the nearby Tunnel Hill Trail, a 45-mile hike-and-bike trail stretching from Harrisburg to White Hill along abandoned railroad beds. There are various access points, but the 9.3-mile section from Tunnel Hill to Vienna is perhaps the most scenic and has several unique features, including the 543-foot tunnel and the longest and highest trestle on the trail. From Ferne Clyffe, go 0.5 miles north on IL 37 to Tunnel Hill Road, then drive 8 miles east. Check **www.dnr.state.il.us/lands/landmgt/parks/r5/tunnel .htm** or call (618) 658-2168 for more information.

GETTING THERE

From I-57, take Exit 40 east, then go 4 miles on CR 13 to Goreville. Turn right on IL 37 and follow it 1.5 miles south to the park entrance, on the left.

From I-24, take Exit 7 west to IL 37 in Goreville and turn left. Go 1.5 miles south to the park entrance, on the left.

GPS COORDINATES

UTM Zone 16S
Easting 0326272
Northing 4155753
Latitude N 37° 31' 56.6649"
Longitude W 88° 57' 58.3844"

44
RED BUD CAMPGROUND/BELL SMITH SPRINGS RECREATION AREA

RED BUD IS A SMALL, QUIET, primitive campground in Bell Smith Springs Recreation Area, off a gravel road in the Shawnee National Forest. It's a great place for a relaxed getaway—but an even better base camp for exploring all the nearby superlative sites in the central Shawnee. Clustered within a few miles of this campground you'll find Illinois' highest waterfall, tallest natural arch, and largest sandstone cave, all within what some consider the most beautiful part of the Shawnee.

At you turn off McCormick Road toward Bell Smith Springs, you'll see a gated drive on the right. That's Teal Pond, formerly a campground but no longer maintained as such by the Forest Service. You can still fish there, but you'll have to hike the short distance past the gate to the three-acre pond.

Two miles farther down the road you'll come to the campground entrance, on the right. Red Bud Campground consists of a single loop with 21 well-shaded sites, each with a table, a fire ring, and a lantern post. Every site is large enough for a tent or two—I prefer sites 3 and 17 for space and shade. Though the sites aren't real isolated from one another, the campground is usually not too busy. When I was there on a beautiful Saturday in June, only two sites were occupied. Take your pick of spots, set up camp, and pay at the self-registration post at the campground entrance.

Drive down the road just a short distance, and you'll come to the main trailhead parking for Bell Smith Springs, one of the most scenic areas in the entire Shawnee Forest. Here four creeks come together in a landscape of canyons, pools, boulders, and shelter caves. This area can be busy, at least on weekends, so plan to hike midweek if possible, or first thing in the morning. Three interconnecting loop trails begin here, and the fourth can be accessed from one of the others.

> *This quiet little campground is a perfect base camp for exploring the superlative sites in the central Shawnee Forest.*

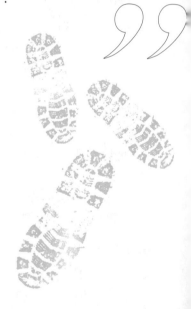

RATINGS

Beauty: ✩ ✩ ✩ ✩ ✩
Privacy: ✩ ✩ ✩
Spaciousness: ✩ ✩ ✩
Quiet: ✩ ✩ ✩ ✩ ✩
Security: ✩ ✩ ✩ ✩
Cleanliness: ✩ ✩ ✩ ✩

ADDRESS:	c/o Vienna/Elizabethtown Ranger District, 602 North First Street, Vienna, IL 62995
OPERATED BY:	U.S. Forest Service
CONTACT:	(618) 658-2111, www.fs.fed.us/r9/ forests/shawnee/ recreation/ camping/redbud
OPEN:	Mar. 15–Dec. 15
SITES:	21
EACH SITE:	Picnic table, fire ring, and lantern pole
ASSIGNMENT:	First come, first served
REGISTRATION:	Self-registration post at entrance
FACILITIES:	Water spigot, vault toilets
PARKING:	At site
FEE:	$10 per night
ELEVATION:	627 feet
RESTRICTIONS:	*Pets:* On leash only *Fires:* In fire rings only *Alcohol:* Permitted *Vehicles:* 2 per site *Other:* 14-day limit; 8 campers per site

Each is marked with color-coded diamonds, totaling about 8 miles of moderately rugged hiking. Particularly in the spring, you will be fording creeks on slippery sandstone, so wear appropriate shoes. You'll find a trail map on the board at the parking area, but it's helpful to have a printed copy, too—you can find one online at **www.fs.fed.us/r9/forests/shawnee/recreation/rogs/maps/bellsmith.jpg.**

Natural Bridge Trail, blazed in yellow, is a 1.5-mile loop that will take you above and below an impressive sandstone arch, 30 feet high and 125 feet long, the highest in the Shawnee Forest. You can climb to the top via the iron rungs anchored to the vertical face (installed back in the 1930s—be careful, one rung is loose!), or take the more circuitous and somewhat safer trail. The blue-blazed 3.2-mile Sentry Bluff loop leads along the cliff edge and down into the canyon to Boulder Falls. Parts of this trail toward the east end of the canyon are rugged and steep, so be prepared for a workout. It runs with Natural Bridge Trail at first, and the two can be combined. White diamonds mark the 1.4-mile General Trail, which leads past the Devil's Backbone ridge, by clear spring-fed pools where some are inclined to take a dip on a hot summer day, and eventually to the spring itself. The 2-mile Mill Branch loop follows the creek canyon of the same name. It's blazed in orange and can be picked up from the end of the white trail or from the Hunting Branch Picnic Area (the first road right before the campground).

Illinois' highest waterfall, Burden Falls, is just 4 miles from the campground, in the Burden Falls Wilderness. Head back up to McCormick Road, turn left, drive 1.5 miles, turn right, and go 0.5 miles to the Burden Falls parking area. There's a smaller set of falls visible from the road, but the 100-foot falls are just a short hike from there. The water flow is very impressive in the spring. A 3.5-mile loop trail begins at the top of the falls, though you may want to get a topographic map before exploring it.

From the highest waterfall, you can head to the country's largest sandstone cave, Sand Cave. Turn left onto McCormick Road and drive 1.9 miles to Cedar Grove Road. Turn right, go 2.4 miles, and turn left just

MAP

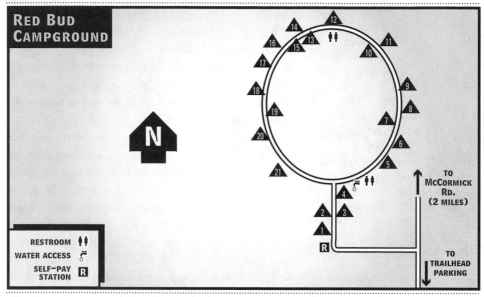

RED BUD CAMPGROUND

N

TO McCORMICK RD. (2 MILES)

RESTROOM
WATER ACCESS
SELF-PAY STATION R

TO TRAILHEAD PARKING

past Cedar Grove Church. Travel 0.2 miles to where you can park by the Forest Service sign. From there a 1-mile well-defined trail leads to the cave, which is about 100 feet long and 30 feet high.

And not far from Bell Smith Springs is the beautiful and rugged Jackson Hollow, the rock climber's mecca at Jackson Falls, the 100-foot cliffs of Indian Kitchen at Lusk Creek Canyon, and Millstone Bluff, with its fascinating remains of a Native American settlement. And there's more! Get a trail map or Susan Post's *Hiking Illinois,* mentioned in Appendix A, and explore.

GETTING THERE

From IL 45, turn east onto CR 8 (Ozark Road), which will become McCormick Road, and watch for Bell Smith Springs signs. Drive 8.5 miles, turn right at the sign, go 1.6 miles, turn right at the next sign, then continue 2 miles to the campground entrance, on the left.

GPS COORDINATES

UTM Zone 16S
Easting 0353555
Northing 4154025
Latitude N 37° 31' 17.6733"
Longitude W 88° 39' 25.9817"

> *If the kids want to do something rather than just enjoy nature, you've got some great options at Dixon Springs.*

DIXON SPRINGS HAS LONG BEEN A PLACE to welcome visitors. More than a century ago, there was a small community, with a post office, gristmill, and general store here. Later a resort developed, complete with a hotel and cabins, and people came from Illinois and neighboring states to take advantage of the purported medicinal benefits of the seven springs for which the town was named. The springs are no longer a prime attraction, but the park and surrounding area still offer lots to see and do, along with a separate, peaceful tent-camping area.

As you enter Dixon Springs off IL 146, go straight, make the second right, and head up the hill, following the signs for tent camping. The road turns right at three historic church buildings and then comes to a picnic pavilion, where you'll find parking for the walk-in tent area. Park staff are rightly proud of this recent addition, which has ten nice sites scattered throughout a wooded area. Most are shaded by tall pines, and you can pitch your tent on a carpet of pine needles. Unlike many parks, which have a few sites dispersed in an open area, at Dixon Springs at least some of the sites are separated from one another by stands of trees and brush. All are considered walk-in sites, but you can actually park your car right next to site 1; site 9, the farthest, is only 215 feet from the lot.

Just off the parking lot, to the right, you'll see a trail with a yellow gate that allows walk-in access to most of the sites. The ones to the left of the trail (sites 1 through 8) are under pine trees. Site 5 is my favorite because it's set back from the others and surrounded by trees so you won't be disturbed by other campers hiking through or around your campsite to reach theirs. Sites 9 and 10 are in deciduous woods; 9 is especially private. Sites 1 through 4 are close to parking—great, as long as you're not sharing the campground with too

RATINGS

Beauty: ✿ ✿ ✿ ✿ ✿
Privacy: ✿ ✿ ✿ ✿
Spaciousness: ✿ ✿ ✿
Quiet: ✿ ✿ ✿ ✿
Security: ✿ ✿ ✿ ✿
Cleanliness: ✿ ✿ ✿ ✿

many other parties. And more often than not, you won't be. On an average non-holiday weekend, only three or four sites will be occupied.

There are vault toilets beyond the campsites and a water spigot and toilets next to the pavilion by the parking lot. The showers are by the swimming pool—check with the park staff or the campground host in the RV section for information.

If you want electricity, there is a separate Class B campground with 39 sites. For groups of up to 80 people, there are six dorm cabins with a kitchen and shower house that can be reserved; they're *very* popular—call January 1 at 7 a.m. to reserve a weekend for that year!

If you've ever taken kids camping and found they want to *do* something rather than just sit around and enjoy nature, you've got some great options at Dixon Springs. They will love the pool with the 45-foot water slide and wading pool for the little ones, and there's a snack bar with sweets and sandwiches. It's open 11 a.m. to 6 p.m. daily, Memorial Day to Labor Day. In 2008 it cost $4 for the whole day, with kids under age 3 free. A private concessionaire operates the pool; call (618) 949-3871 for current information.

Before swimming, you and the kids can get a little nature in with a hike on Ghost Dance Canyon Trail, which starts right by the pool parking lot. The name alone is sure to pique their interest, and the canyon will hold it. The trail winds between canyon walls as high as 60 feet, following a rippling creek past a waterfall and huge stands of boulders that beg to be explored. The trail itself is 1 mile long, but the canyon continues, and you can push farther without fear of getting lost. Bring a camera—you'll want to get photos of some of the unique rock formations and perhaps a shot of the kids perched atop a mound of boulders like conquering heroes.

Just 3 miles north of Dixon Springs, on IL 145, is Lake Glendale, with boating, fishing, and a public beach. And if you have an archaeological bent, head 5 miles farther north to Millstone Bluff, the remains of a prehistoric Native American settlement perched on a cliff rising 320 feet above the surrounding terrain. A 0.5-mile trail takes you past the remains of the cemetery and a village that was probably last occupied around

KEY INFORMATION

ADDRESS:	RR 2, Box 178, Route 146, Golconda, IL 62938
OPERATED BY:	IDNR
CONTACT:	(618) 949-3394, www.dnr.state.il.us/lands/land mgt/parks/r5/dixon.htm
OPEN:	Year-round
SITES:	Class D: 10 walk-in tent sites; Class B: 39 sites
EACH SITE:	Picnic table, fire ring; only Class B has electric
ASSIGNMENT:	First come, first served
REGISTRATION:	Set up first, then register at office
FACILITIES:	Water spigots, vault toilets, showers; swimming pool available for fee
PARKING:	Class B: at site; Class D: in lot
FEE:	Class B: $18 per night; Class D: $6 per night
ELEVATION:	507 feet
RESTRICTIONS:	*Pets:* On leash only *Fires:* In fire rings only *Alcohol:* Permitted *Vehicles:* 2 per site *Other:* 14-day limit; 1 RV and 1 tent, or 2 tents per site; 4 adults or 1 family per site

MAP

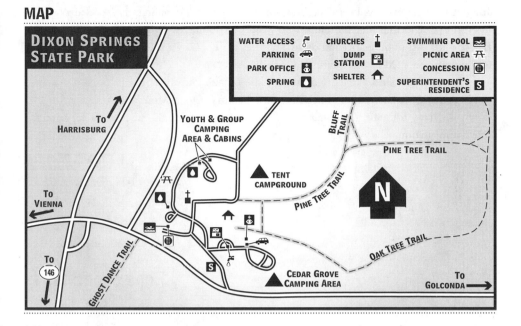

DIXON SPRINGS STATE PARK

WATER ACCESS	CHURCHES	SWIMMING POOL
PARKING	DUMP STATION	PICNIC AREA
PARK OFFICE	SHELTER	CONCESSION
SPRING		SUPERINTENDENT'S RESIDENCE

To HARRISBURG

To VIENNA

To 146

YOUTH & GROUP CAMPING AREA & CABINS

TENT CAMPGROUND

BLUFF TRAIL

PINE TREE TRAIL

PINE TREE TRAIL

OAK TREE TRAIL

GHOST DANCE TRAIL

CEDAR GROVE CAMPING AREA

To GOLCONDA

MAP

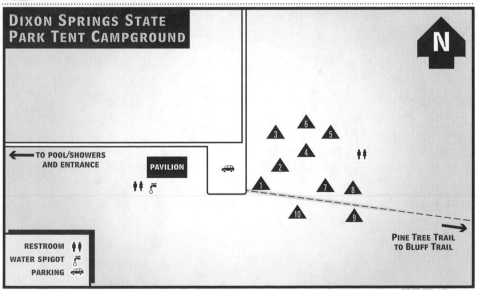

DIXON SPRINGS STATE PARK TENT CAMPGROUND

TO POOL/SHOWERS AND ENTRANCE

PAVILION

PINE TREE TRAIL TO BLUFF TRAIL

RESTROOM	
WATER SPIGOT	
PARKING	

1500 A.D. There isn't a lot to see, but you may find it fascinating, as I do, to read the interpretive signs and imagine those who lived there some 500 years ago. Head north on IL 145—just east of the park—and drive 5.5 miles to IL 147. Turn left (west), and go 1 mile to the entrance to Millstone Bluff, on the right.

And at least stop and be tempted by the amazing array of confections just across the highway from the park at The Chocolate Factory. Open Monday through Saturday, they also have fountain drinks and ice cream. Check **www.thechocolatefactory.net** for more information.

GETTING THERE

From I-24, take Exit 16 at
Vienna to access IL 146 East.
Go 12 miles to the park
entrance, on the left.

GPS COORDINATES

UTM Zone 16S
Easting 0352495
Northing 4138379
Latitude N 37° 22' 49.5780"
Longitude W 88° 39' 57.8936"

A little fishing, a little hiking, a little relaxation as you camp next to the lake—these are good reasons for selecting Saline County.

A **LITTLE FISHING, A LITTLE HIKING,** a little relaxation as you camp next to the lakeshore, plus proximity to the Shawnee Forest—these are good reasons for selecting Saline County Fish & Wildlife Area for a camping getaway. The 1,200-plus acres around Glen O. Jones Lake were once known for their salt springs (hence the county's name); today they serve as a recreational destination.

The campsites at Saline County are not concentrated in one place you could call "the campground" but rather are spread out along the rectangular loop of the main park road. Each site has a ground grill, a table, and a lantern pole; water spigots and vault toilets are nearby. Sites 1 through 23 face the lake on the south side of the loop, while sites 25 through 43 are on the north side, in grassy fields surrounded by woods. As you enter the park from the south, pass the road to the park office and head left at the fork. You'll pass the concession (closed in summer 2008), then the campground host, where you can register after you've selected your site. Sites 1 through 12 are the first you come to along the lakeshore. These are smaller, closer together, and popular but certainly offer a beautiful view of the lake. If you want one of these, site 4 would be my choice for space.

Sites 13 and 14 are on the southwest corner of the loop, and to the left is a parking lot for sites 15 through 23. These are also on the lake, and also popular, but if you want to fish or camp near water, this is the place to be. Site 19 is a bit bigger and is next to a floating dock— good for fishing, but by far the best lakefront site is 23—flat, shaded, spacious, and all by itself on a point extending into the lake.

Up the hill and to the right are sites 25 through 43. Here you can spread out a bit more than down by the lake—sites are fairly spacious and level. They are grouped

RATINGS

Beauty: ✪ ✪ ✪
Privacy: ✪ ✪ ✪
Spaciousness: ✪ ✪ ✪
Quiet: ✪ ✪ ✪
Security: ✪ ✪ ✪ ✪ ✪
Cleanliness: ✪ ✪ ✪ ✪

in sections along the road: sites 25 through 32 are together, then 33 through 35, then 36 through 39. Since these are not as popular as the lakefront sites, select a site in one of the latter two sections and you may end up with no campers nearby. The last four sites, 40 through 43, occupy a secluded wooded loop in the northeast corner of the park. This is labeled the equestrian area but isn't limited to campers with horses. However, park staff will tell you it's informally known as "the party area"—this is where groups that want to stay up later and be a little louder come to camp. If that's not you, this is probably an area to avoid on the weekends. Midweek or off-season, though, it should be a perfect place for privacy. Camping normally fills up only on holiday weekends—on any other fair-weather weekend, about half to two-thirds of the sites will be occupied.

Fishing is good at Saline County. You can bank or boat fish on 105-acre Glen O. Jones Lake for large-mouth bass, bluegill, redear, crappie, and channel catfish. There are two launching ramps and two docks, and if the state can contract with another concessionaire, there will be boat rentals again. You can also go after trout on the two-acre trout pond stocked annually with rainbow trout.

For hiking, there are four trails in the park. Lake Trail is 3 miles long, traveling around the lake from the dam to site 13. River Trail is 1 mile long, heading from the equestrian campground through woods down to the Saline River. Wildlife Nature Trail is a short, easy 0.75-mile loop in the middle of the park. Cave Hill Trail begins in the northwest corner of the park loop, by the bronze statue of Tecumseh. This is a more rugged 3-mile trail that ascends along a ridge with ravines on either side and climbs to Cave Hill, offering some excellent views of the surrounding countryside. It also leads to Equality Cave. However, the cave itself is gated by the Forest Service and closed for at least the next couple of years to protect a bat species rare to the area. It may reopen seasonally, by permit, but if you're looking for a first "wild cave" to explore, Equality isn't a good choice. Even locals have gotten lost in this maze of a cave before.

Just 6 miles from Saline County is another of the Shawnee National Forest's many interesting sandstone

ADDRESS: 85 Glen O. Jones Road, Equality, IL 62934

OPERATED BY: IDNR

CONTACT: (618) 276-4405, www.dnr.state.il.us/lands/landmgt/parks/r5/saline.htm

OPEN: Year-round

SITES: Class C: 43 sites

EACH SITE: Picnic tables, fire pit and grill, lantern post

ASSIGNMENT: First come, first served

REGISTRATION: Register with campground host (if available) or set up and park staff will come by

FACILITIES: Water spigots, vault toilets

PARKING: At site

FEE: $8 per night

ELEVATION: 381 feet

RESTRICTIONS: *Pets:* On leash only
Fires: In fire rings only
Alcohol: Permitted
Vehicles: 2 per site
Other: 14-day limit; 1 RV and 1 tent, or 2 tents per site; 2 families per site

MAP

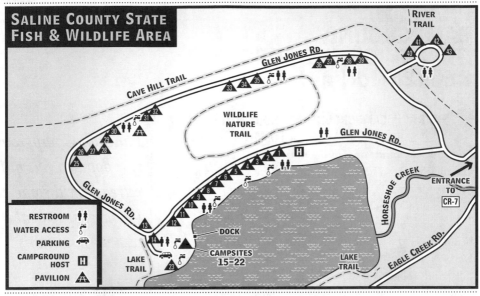

SALINE COUNTY STATE FISH & WILDLIFE AREA

RIVER TRAIL

GLEN JONES RD.

CAVE HILL TRAIL

WILDLIFE NATURE TRAIL

GLEN JONES RD.

GLEN JONES RD.

HORSESHOE CREEK

ENTRANCE TO CR-7

ENTRANCE TO CR-7

Eagle Creek Rd.

DOCK

CAMPSITES 15-22

LAKE TRAIL

LAKE TRAIL

RESTROOM	👫
WATER ACCESS	💧
PARKING	🚗
CAMPGROUND HOST	H
PAVILION	▲

GETTING THERE

From US 45 in Harrisburg, drive east 9.5 miles on IL 13 to IL 142 at Equality. Turn right. Go 1 mile, then turn right at the brown park sign onto Walnut Street/CR 7. Follow the signs 4.5 miles to the left turn onto CR 15, then drive 0.5 miles to the park entrance, on the left.

formations: Stone Face, which resembles, as you might expect, the side profile of a man's head. The moderately rugged loop trail to Stone Face is about 1.75 miles long and leads past a shelter cave and some impressive bluff views. From the Saline County exit, turn left, go 0.5 miles north to CR 17, and turn left. Go 3 miles on CR 17 to Stoneface Road and turn left. Continue 1.75 miles south on Stoneface Road to the entrance, on the left.

GPS COORDINATES

UTM Zone 16S
Easting 0378539
Northing 4172487
Latitude N 37° 41' 29.6268"
Longitude W 88° 22' 39.4907"

PHARAOH CAMPGROUND/ GARDEN OF THE GODS RECREATION AREA

PHARAOH CAMPGROUND AT GARDEN OF THE **GODS** Recreation Area is a popular but quiet retreat amid some of the most spectacular scenery in Illinois. Whether you camp there or just visit for the day while staying elsewhere, Garden of the Gods is a must-see.

The drive to Garden of the Gods is almost as beautiful as the destination itself. It is located along Karbers Ridge Road, which snakes among wooded hills and rolling meadows as it passes through the Shawnee National Forest. Whether you pick up Karbers Ridge off IL 1 to the east or IL 34 to the west, take your time and enjoy the scenery.

Turn north off Karbers Ridge Road at the Garden of the Gods sign, and go about 1.4 miles to the left turn into the recreation area. Another 1.4 miles brings you to a T-intersection—take a left for trailhead parking, or a right for the campground.

Pharaoh Campground consists of a single loop with 12 sites on its south side. Each has a fire ring, picnic table, and lantern pole. There's a set of vault toilets next to site 6, and a hand-operated water pump at the loop entrance. Most sites enjoy the shade of tall, stately pines, and some offer a panoramic view of the valley below and the Shawnee Hills. Sites 2 and 10 are well shaded, and 12 offers the most space and seclusion, being at the end. Sites 7 and 9 have the best views, and site 7 has trees on either side, separating it from the adjacent sites.

The most impressive thing about Pharaoh is the quiet. Even some of the most secluded campgrounds I've visited are often close enough to a highway, railway, or just the road through the park that some mechanized noise is inevitable. Not so here. Pharaoh is in the middle of a wilderness area, perched high above the valley, far from any transportation clamor. To be sure, the trailhead parking down on the other side of

> *Pharaoh Campground is a popular but quiet retreat amid some of the most spectacular scenery in Illinois.*

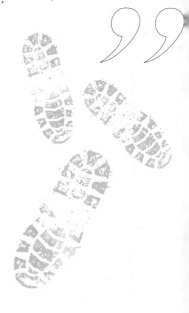

RATINGS

Beauty: ✩ ✩ ✩ ✩ ✩
Privacy: ✩ ✩ ✩
Spaciousness: ✩ ✩ ✩
Quiet: ✩ ✩ ✩ ✩ ✩
Security: ✩ ✩ ✩ ✩
Cleanliness: ✩ ✩ ✩ ✩

KEY INFORMATION

ADDRESS:	c/o Hidden Springs Ranger District, 602 North First Street, Vienna, IL 62995
OPERATED BY:	U.S. Forest Service
CONTACT:	(618) 658-2111, www.fs.fed.us/r9/ forests/shawnee/ recreation/camp ing/pharaoh
OPEN:	Year-round
SITES:	12 tent sites
EACH SITE:	Picnic table, fire ring, and lantern pole
ASSIGNMENT:	First come, first served
REGISTRATION:	Self-registration post at entrance
FACILITIES:	Hand pump, vault toilets
PARKING:	At site
FEE:	$10 per night
ELEVATION:	845 feet
RESTRICTIONS:	*Pets:* On leash only *Fires:* In fire rings only *Alcohol:* Permitted *Vehicles:* 2 per site *Other:* 14-day limit; 8 campers per site

the T-intersection is very busy, especially on weekends. Garden of the Gods is the most-visited site in the Shawnee National Forest. But that doesn't affect the campground. And though the campground will be nearly full on most fair-weather weekends, the people who camp at Pharaoh are not usually partiers but hikers and backpackers who appreciate and guard the stillness.

If you are fortunate enough to have a clear sky at night at Pharaoh, you can enjoy stargazing as well. With the relatively high altitude (830 feet) and the lack of city lights nearby, the nighttime celestial vistas are as stunning as the daytime terrestrial ones.

At some point during your stay at Pharaoh, you will hike the 0.25-mile Observation Trail. Stroll down the hill to the parking area and trail entrance. Bring drinking water in a non-disposable container (disposables are not permitted). The trail is paved but steep in places, and you'll want good hiking shoes so you can safely clamber up, over, and around these amazing sandstone formations. Be careful near the bluffs and hang on to small children. The sign at the trailhead says to allow 45 minutes, but you may want to spend much longer simply sitting and enjoying the breathtaking views. Bring a camera to snap a picture of Camel Rock, probably the most-photographed natural feature in Illinois.

To see more of the geological wonders of the area, take the trailhead starting at the north end of the parking area. Go 0.2 miles north to the trail junction on the left past Anvil Rock. Turn left (west), and at the next trail junction you can go right (north) or left (south). Going right about 0.5 miles takes you first to Mushroom Rock, and then to the Noah's Ark formation. Head left to pass Shelter Rock and other formations. At 0.6 miles you'll reach the River-to-River Trail. Here take the trail marked "Lower Trail." You pass beneath all the formations seen from the Observation Trail. After 0.5 miles you'll cross the park road. Follow the trail as it circles the bluffs below the camping area. At 0.75 miles from the road, you'll reach another trail junction on the left. Make the left and climb 0.25 miles to the campground road. These trails are normally well signed, but it's wise to bring a trail map just in case. A useful one can be found at **cewalter.tripod.com/id26.htm.**

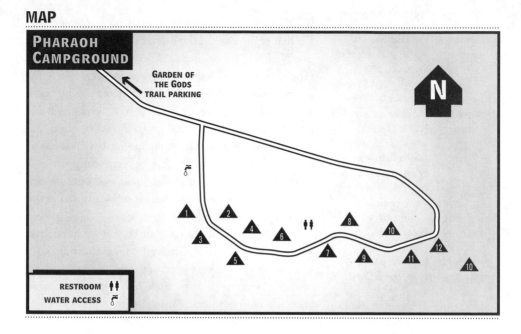

If you want to visit Garden of the Gods but would rather camp some place less busy, try Camp Cadiz—head 3 miles east on Karbers Ridge Road, take a right on Cadiz Road, then go 3.7 miles. If you'd like a campground with a swimming beach, check out Pine Ridge at the Pounds Hollow Recreation Area, 6.6 miles east on Karbers Ridge Road.

GETTING THERE

From Harrisburg, take IL 34 south 15.3 miles to Karbers Ridge Road. Turn left and go 2.8 miles to the Garden of the Gods sign at CR 10. Make another left and proceed 1.4 miles north to the entrance, on the left. From IL 1, turn west onto CR 13/Pounds Hollow Road. Go 8.5 miles (this becomes Karbers Ridge Road) to the sign at CR 10, turn right, and drive 1.4 miles north to the entrance, on the left.

GPS COORDINATES

UTM Zone 16S
Easting 0379376
Northing 4162394
Latitude N 37° 36' 2.6016"
Longitude W 88° 21' 59.3542"

> *Pine Ridge is an underappreciated gem, where you can camp in a beautiful pine wood near a tranquil beach.*

PINE RIDGE CAMPGROUND IN THE Pounds Hollow Recreation Area has to be one of the most underappreciated camping gems in southern Illinois. While it officially has 75 sites, half of these are closed most of the time, opened as overflow only on the busier Memorial Day and Labor Day weekends, and even then they're not necessary. Since Pine Ridge has no electric sites and no shower, it's not popular with the modern RV crowd. A fair-weather non-holiday weekend may only see five to ten sites occupied—which is all the better for those of us who don't mind tent camping in a beautiful pine wood, near a tranquil beach, great hiking, and all the attractions of the eastern Shawnee National Forest.

As you enter the recreation area, take the left fork to go to the campground. Pass the two closed camping loops, containing sites 1 through 13, and 14 through 35. You'll come to the first open camping spur off to the left, with sites 54 through 76, and then a little farther on, the spur with sites 36 through 53.

As the name suggests, all the sites are nicely shaded under stately, tall pines. Each has a table, a ground grill, and a lantern pole, and sufficient room for a tent or two. They aren't far apart, but since the campground is rarely busy, you should find plenty of privacy. I prefer the spur containing sites 36 through 53, where the sites are more spacious. Sites 46, 47, and 48, toward the end of the spur, are good choices. In the other section, I like 56, 61, 73, and 75 for shade and space. Unlike at some campgrounds, the sites in the loops at the end of the road are smaller and not as good. There are vault toilets in both spurs, but the only water spigot is toward the end of the first, near site 65.

Once you've selected your site, as with all campgrounds in the Shawnee National Forest, return to the

RATINGS

Beauty: ✪ ✪ ✪ ✪
Privacy: ✪ ✪ ✪ ✪
Spaciousness: ✪ ✪
Quiet: ✪ ✪ ✪ ✪ ✪
Security: ✪ ✪ ✪ ✪
Cleanliness: ✪ ✪ ✪ ✪

campground entrance to register and pay at the self-registration post.

Back at the recreation-area entrance, take the right fork, and you'll be on the one-way loop headed to Pounds Hollow Lake and a very picturesque and quiet beach. The beach area was first constructed in 1938 by the Civilian Conservation Corps, and their excellent work can still be seen in the hand-cut sandstone foundation of the picnic shelter. It has recently been refurbished, and now has a beautiful picnic area, changing rooms, flush toilets, a cold-water "shower tower" on the beach, and some nice fishing areas off to the north side. It's not a big beach, but it's usually not crowded—and it's free!

I enjoy a day of warming up with hiking in the morning and cooling off with swimming in the afternoon, and Pounds Hollow makes that easy. At the end of the beach is part of Beaver Trail, which leads to the canyons, shelter caves, and an overlook of Rim Rock Recreation Trail. You'll reach Rim Rock in just 0.5 miles and can explore the cool canyons below. Be sure to check out Ox-Lot Cave, a historic shelter bluff cave. Climb the stairway to the 0.8-mile loop trail above, where you'll see the remnants of a Native American wall, and look out over Pounds Hollow Lake. Near the stairwell is "Fat Man's Misery," where you can squeeze through huge boulders. The trail is well marked and designated "hiker-only" for this portion, so you won't be sharing it with horses. Water and toilets are available at the Rim Rock parking area, off the loop trail above.

You can also hike Beaver Trail in the other direction, starting from the earthen dam at the north end of the lake. The trail runs a total of 9 miles to Camp Cadiz, but the most interesting portion is the first mile, to Karbers Ridge Road; you'll go up and down hills, past creeks, and by rocky outcrops.

If Pine Ridge suits you as a base camp, you can, in fact, explore much of the eastern Shawnee Forest from there. Pounds Hollow is conveniently close to the must-see Garden of the Gods. From the park entrance, go 6.6 miles west on Karbers Ridge Road, then head 1.4 miles north. (See the Pharaoh Campground profile for more details.) Even closer, though, is the less famous High Knob, a 929-foot sandstone prominence with a

KEY INFORMATION

ADDRESS:	c/o Vienna/Elizabethtown Ranger District, 602 North First Street, Vienna, IL 62995
OPERATED BY:	US Forest Service
CONTACT:	(618) 658-2111, www.fs.fed.us/r9/ forests/shawnee/ recreation/camping/pineridge
OPEN:	Apr. 1–Dec. 15
SITES:	35
EACH SITE:	Picnic table, fire ring, and lantern pole
ASSIGNMENT:	First come, first served
REGISTRATION:	Self-registration post at entrance
FACILITIES:	Water spigot, vault toilets
PARKING:	At site
FEE:	$10 per night
ELEVATION:	651 feet
RESTRICTIONS:	*Pets:* On leash only *Fires:* In fire rings only *Alcohol:* Permitted *Vehicles:* 2 per site *Other:* 14-day limit; 8 campers per site

MAP

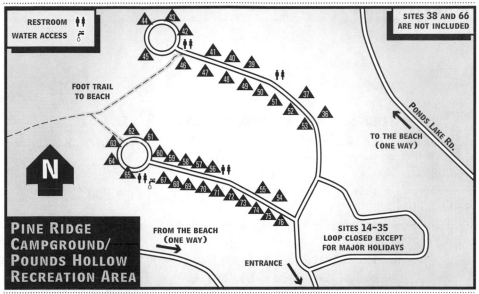

RESTROOM
WATER ACCESS

SITES 38 AND 66
ARE NOT INCLUDED

FOOT TRAIL
TO BEACH

PONDS LAKE RD.

TO THE BEACH
(ONE WAY)

N

PINE RIDGE
CAMPGROUND/
POUNDS HOLLOW
RECREATION AREA

FROM THE BEACH
(ONE WAY)

SITES 14–35
LOOP CLOSED EXCEPT
FOR MAJOR HOLIDAYS

ENTRANCE

GETTING THERE

From Harrisburg, take IL 34 south 15.3 miles to Karbers Ridge Road. Turn left and go 9.5 miles (this becomes Pounds Hollow Road at about 8 miles) to the Pounds Hollow sign. Turn left. From IL 1, turn west onto CR 13/Pounds Hollow Road. Drive 1.9 miles to the Pounds Hollow sign and turn right.

2-mile loop trail and some excellent views. Travel 5 miles west of Pounds Hollow on Karbers Ridge Road, then 1.6 miles north on CR 2 to Knob Hill. Make a right about 0.8 miles up the hill and pass the horse camp to reach the High Knob picnic area.

GPS COORDINATES

UTM Zone 16S
Easting 0388149
Northing 4163531
Latitude N 37° 36' 43.5029"
Longitude W 88° 16' 2.2745"

49
CAMP CADIZ

THE EASTERN SHAWNEE NATIONAL FOREST boasts some great places for tent campers. Pharaoh Campground at Garden of the Gods is well known for its scenery, Pine Ridge for its beach, and Red Bud for the canyons and streams of nearby Bell Smith Springs.

The Shawnee's easternmost campground, Camp Cadiz, can't offer any of that. What it does offer, however, is your best chance in the whole Shawnee Forest to camp at an established campground with no one else around. If you're seeking solitude but still like the convenience of your car, a toilet, and water nearby, Camp Cadiz is a good choice just about any time outside deer-hunting season. You may, on occasion, find a neighbor or two camping, but chances are they'll be just as eager for quiet as you are.

As you're coming down Cadiz Road, watch for the old chimneys on the left, the last remnants of the Civilian Conservation Corps camp that once stood here. Turn left, and you'll find the signboard and self-registration post at the entrance to the campground loop. Going counter-clockwise around the loop are sites 1 to 11, each with a fire ring, picnic table, and lantern pole. Site 1, on the outside of the loop at the first chimney, has no shade and, like sites 3 and 5, is too close to the gravel road. Not much traffic passes here, but you might as well be farthest from it. Sites 2, 4, and 6, inside the loop, are grass-covered and somewhat shaded. Sites 7 and 8 are by the vault toilets and water spigot. The best sites are 9, 10, and 11, at the back of the loop; 9 is my favorite because it's at the edge of the woods. Note that you may rarely see equestrians camping here.

When I was at Camp Cadiz, the water spigot was broken (it was fixed later in the season), and some sites needed mowing. Forest Service personnel keep up with maintenance as best they can, but the Shawnee is vast

> *If you're seeking solitude, Camp Cadiz is a good choice.*

RATINGS

Beauty: ✩ ✩ ✩
Privacy: ✩ ✩ ✩
Spaciousness: ✩ ✩ ✩
Quiet: ✩ ✩ ✩ ✩ ✩
Security: ✩ ✩ ✩
Cleanliness: ✩ ✩ ✩ ✩

ADDRESS:	c/o Hidden Springs Ranger District, 602 North First Street, Vienna, IL 62995
OPERATED BY:	US Forest Service
CONTACT:	(618) 658-2111, www.fs.fed.us/r9/ forests/shawnee/ recreation/ camping/cadiz
OPEN:	Apr. 1–Dec. 15
SITES:	11 tent sites
EACH SITE:	Picnic table, fire ring, and lantern pole
ASSIGNMENT:	First come, first served
REGISTRATION:	Self-registration post at entrance
FACILITIES:	Vault toilets, water spigot
PARKING:	At site
FEE:	$10 per night
ELEVATION:	599 feet
RESTRICTIONS:	*Pets:* On leash only *Fires:* In fire rings only *Alcohol:* Permitted *Vehicles:* 2 per site *Other:* 14-day limit; 2 tents and 8 campers per site

and staff few. Some repairs and even routine upkeep can be delayed, particularly at a little-visited site like Camp Cadiz. This is one campground where you'd be wise to bring drinking water and even toilet paper, just in case. You can also check the Shawnee National Forest's homepage before coming (**www.fs.fed.us/r9/forests/ shawnee**); there you'll find regularly updated information about closings and changes in available services.

Camp Cadiz is a trailhead for the River-to-River Trail, which runs approximately 160 miles (or more, depending on who's measuring) across southern Illinois, from Battery Rock on the Ohio River in the east, to Devil's Backbone on the Mississippi to the west. Back-packers who use Camp Cadiz as a starting point can park on the grass opposite sites 7 and 8. If you're not up to the whole multi-week trek, there are, fortunately, more than 20 trailheads along it where you can park and day hike specific sections. If you have a hiking partner with a second vehicle, you can shuttle one to your destination, hike, and return in comfort to your campsite, perhaps stopping for a well-earned dinner on the way. From Camp Cadiz you can go south to Rock Creek (about 4 miles), or north to High Knob (about 10 miles—a popular and scenic stretch). Note that you may be sharing the trail with horses and mountain bikers. The River-to-River is generally well blazed—its sign bearing a blue lowercase "i" in a white diamond—but if you plan to hike any portion you should definitely invest in a topographical map and a compass or GPS. The River-to-River Trail Society (**www.rivertorivertrail.com**) publishes the best guide—a new edition is due out in early 2009.

Many visitors to the area hit Garden of the Gods and conclude they've "done" the Shawnee, but whether you hike or drive, go to High Knob, which boasts its own spectacular and less-seen views and rock formations. This rocky prominence sits at 929 feet, with about 2 miles of loop trail circling the base of the cliffs, passing shelter bluffs and traversing slot canyons. Head east on Cadiz Road to Karbers Ridge Road, 5.3 miles from Camp Cadiz. Turn right at the High Knob sign, go 1.7 miles north, and turn right again to reach the parking area. A short trail leads to an overlook; the loop trails begin back down the road a bit.

MAP

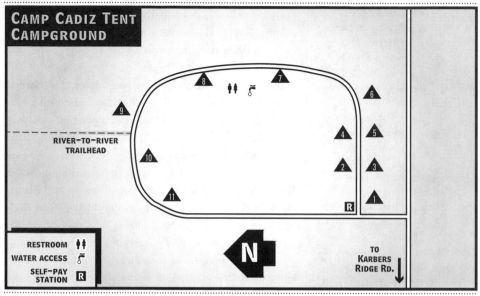

CAMP CADIZ TENT CAMPGROUND

8 7

9

RIVER-TO-RIVER
TRAILHEAD

6

4 5

10

2 3

11

1

R

RESTROOM
WATER ACCESS
SELF-PAY
STATION

N

TO
KARBERS
RIDGE RD.

Not far south or east of Camp Cadiz, you'll find the Ohio River, with its interesting small towns and scenic overlooks. Historic Battery Rock was so named because it served as a fortification during the Civil War. Guns were mounted in the square holes in the rocks, and if you look carefully you'll see names and the date 1861 engraved in the stone. To get there from Camp Cadiz, head east on Cadiz Road to IL 1. Turn right and drive 6.4 miles south to Lamb Road. Turn left and proceed 5.7 miles, going straight at the fork at 4.5 miles, and left at the fork at 5.4 miles.

GETTING THERE

From Harrisburg, take IL 34 south 15.3 miles to Karbers Ridge Road. Turn left and go 9.6 miles east to Camp Cadiz entrance on the left. From the junction of IL 1 and IL 13, go 12.5 miles south on IL 1 to Cadiz Road. Turn right and go 2.8 miles west to Camp Cadiz entrance on the right.

GPS COORDINATES

UTM Zone 16S
Easting 0390066
Northing 4159671
Latitude N 37° 34' 39.1021"
Longitude W 88° 14' 41.9854"

> *Take in the sweeping views of the Ohio River valley from this historic—ande ven notorious—landmark.*

FEW PARKS IN ILLINOIS CAN LAY CLAIM to as much fascinating history and even notoriety as Cave-in-Rock State Park, just east of the town of the same name on the Ohio River. From the 1790s to the 1830s, the 55-foot-wide cave in a bluff overlooking the river served variously as a hideout for counterfeiters, a lair for pirates who preyed on river traffic, and a "Liquor Vault and House of Entertainment." The cave itself is equally intriguing, and this is one place in southern Illinois where you're sure to see flocks of tourists during the summer. Fortunately, most don't spend the night, so the campground, while popular, is not nearly so crowded.

As you enter the park, take the first left. You'll enter the Class A section of the campground, a large loop of 34 electric sites with plenty of grassy space but not much shade. Many sites have ample room for tents, but RVs predominate, and most weekends this area will be at least three-quarters full. Continue right around the circle, and take the next right uphill to the entrance to the tent-camping area. Sixteen non-electric sites lie along two spurs: sites 1 through 6 are on the left, and 7 through 16 are on the right. All sites have a ground grill and table; there are water and vault toilets at the tent-area entrance. Additionally, all campers can use the shower house in the Class A section. Sites here are smaller but better shaded, and this area isn't as busy—perhaps half full on non-holiday weekends.

The spur to the left is on sloping ground, so I prefer the more level sites to the right. Sites 11, 13, and 14 are nicely shaded, and 16 is a bit farther from the road and other sites. You can go ahead and set up before registering with the campground host at site 1 in the Class A section, or park staff will come by later. Firewood is usually available from the campground host.

RATINGS

Beauty: ☆ ☆ ☆
Privacy: ☆ ☆ ☆
Spaciousness: ☆ ☆ ☆
Quiet: ☆ ☆ ☆
Security: ☆ ☆ ☆ ☆ ☆
Cleanliness: ☆ ☆ ☆ ☆

For those not wanting to rough it, Cave-in-Rock also has four duplex cabins with eight suites altogether. Each suite has two queen beds, a living room, a private bathroom, a refrigerator, and a private deck with unrivalled views of the Ohio River. The small restaurant offers a good selection of breakfast items, sandwiches, and dinners, including all-you-can-eat catfish on Fridays and fried chicken on Sundays.

You'll, of course, want to check out the cave: the short trail begins at the parking area across the road from the campground entrance. Be careful—as you descend the rough stone steps, you'll want to take in the sweeping views of the Ohio River, almost 0.5 miles wide at this point. Although the cave entrance is huge, the cave itself is only about 160 feet deep. A sinkhole in the ceiling forms a natural skylight, so you won't need a flashlight. This is a cool place on a hot summer day. Unlike the sandstone bluff shelters in the Shawnee Forest, this is a solutional cave, formed as water pushed its way out to the river, gradually dissolving the limestone bedrock. At one time the cave was probably much longer, but over thousands of years the Ohio River shaved off its southern end.

Most visitors "do" the cave and leave, missing the hiking trails and opportunities to explore the woods and the park's scenic vistas. Make the most of this park: You can pick up the Hickory Ridge and Pirate's Bluff trails east of the tent campground; together they total about 1.75 miles. There are other unmarked trails along the river and bluffs.

About 4 miles west of the town of Cave-in-Rock, you can get another outstanding view of the river valley from the bluffs at Tower Rock. Head west on Clay Street, which becomes Cave-in-Rock Road, to Tower Rock Road, and turn left. A short trail from the east side of the parking area climbs to the overlook. You can also camp here (no fee, no facilities), but the area is sometimes closed due to flooding. Call the US Forest Service at (618) 658-2111 for current information.

For a different view of the cave and countryside, try a boat trip on the Ohio River. The *Shawnee Queen* river taxi plies the waters between Cave-in-Rock and Golconda Marina, about 26 miles to the west, with

KEY INFORMATION

ADDRESS:	#1 New State Park Road, Box 338, Cave-In-Rock, IL 62919
OPERATED BY:	IDNR
CONTACT:	(618) 289-4325, www.dnr.state.il .us/lands/land mgt/parks/r5/ caverock.htm
OPEN:	Year-round
SITES:	16 Class B sites; 34 Class A sites
EACH SITE:	Picnic table, fire ring and grate; electric (Class A only)
ASSIGNMENT:	First come, first served
REGISTRATION:	Register with host or set up and park staff will come by
FACILITIES:	Water spigots, vault toilets, shower house; lodge with 4 duplex cottages; restaurant
PARKING:	At site
FEE:	Class A: $20 per night, $30 per night holidays; Class B: $10 per night
ELEVATION:	344 feet
RESTRICTIONS:	*Pets:* On leash only *Fires:* In fire rings only *Alcohol:* Permitted *Vehicles:* 4 per site *Other:* 14-day limit; 1 RV and 1 tent, or 4 tents per site

MAP

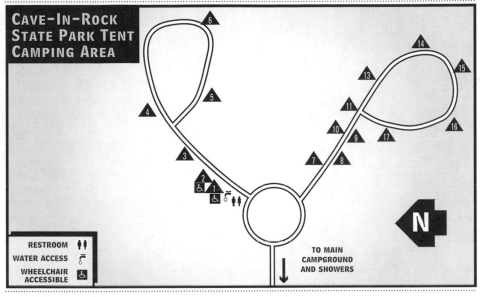

CAVE-IN-ROCK
STATE PARK TENT
CAMPING AREA

RESTROOM
WATER ACCESS
WHEELCHAIR
ACCESSIBLE

TO MAIN
CAMPGROUND
AND SHOWERS

N

GETTING THERE

From I-57 at Marion, take Exit 54 to access IL 13 East. Go 38 miles, through Harrisburg, to IL 1. Turn right and drive 22 miles south to the town of Cave-in-Rock. Turn left at the park sign on Main Street, and head 0.25 miles to the park entrance.

GPS COORDINATES

UTM Zone 16S
Easting 0397224
Northing 4147356
Latitude N 37° 28' 2.5544"
Longitude W 88° 9' 44.0070"

stops at Elizabethtown and Rosiclaire along the way. The trip is certainly scenic and relaxed—or slow, depending on your perspective. It's about two hours one-way, with two round-trips per day, and you can board and disembark at any stop. The *Shawnee Queen* runs from mid-May to November 1, Tuesday through Saturday. Reservations are recommended. Check **www .ridesmtd.com/shawneequeenfares.htm** or call (618) 285-3342 for more information.

If your river journey includes Golconda Marina, pick up a picnic lunch in town and hike or drive up the nearby Rauchfuss Hill. You'll be treated to another panoramic view of the river and probably have the place to yourself. The trail from the marina is a steep 0.5 miles; the entrance by road is 0.5 miles north of the marina on IL 146, to the right. Primitive camping (with water and vault toilets) is normally available, but in 2008 the remnants of Hurricane Ike downed numerous trees. Check with Dixon Springs State Park at (618) 949-3394 for current conditions.

APPENDIX A:
SOURCES OF INFORMATION

The following books and Web sites have been useful and enhanced my travels around Illinois.

BOOKS

Henry, Steve. *60 Hikes Within 60 Miles: St. Louis. 2nd edition*. Birmingham, Alabama: Menasha Ridge Press, 2007.

Villaire, Ted. *60 Hikes Within 60 Miles: Chicago. 2nd edition*. Birmingham, Alabama: Menasha Ridge Press, 2008.
   Titles in the *60 Hikes Within 60 Miles* series contain the most detailed trail descriptions and maps you'll find anywhere. The St. Louis guide includes four hiking venues in Illinois.

Johnsen, David. *Biking Illinois*. Trails Media Group, 2006.
   Detailed maps and trails descriptions covering the state.

Post, Susan L. *Hiking Illinois*. Champaign, Illinois: Human Kinetics, 1997.
   This is my favorite hiking guide for the state as a whole, with detailed descriptions of 100 day hikes, including many around campgrounds I've included.

Ries, Richard and Dave Shepard. *Mountain Bike! Midwest: Ohio, Indiana, and Illinois. 2nd edition*. Birmingham, Alabama: Menasha Ridge Press, 2000.
   Excellent, detailed descriptions and maps of mountain biking trails in the greater Chicago area and Shawnee National Forest, along with Jubilee College, Rock Island Trail, and Kickapoo State Park. This one is currently out of print, but you might be able to locate a copy in a used bookstore or on the Web.

River-to-River Trail Society. *River-to-River Trail Guide. 3rd edition*. Harrisburg, Illinois, 2002.
   The only guide that covers the entire River-to-River Trail in southern Illinois. A new edition is planned for early 2009. Order at www.rivertorivertrail.com or (618) 252-6789.

Svob, Mike. *Paddling Illinois: 64 Great Trips by Canoe and Kayak*. Madison, Wisconsin: Trails Books, 2000.
   Some of the information on outfitters is outdated, but overall the descriptions of waterways and access points are detailed.

Ulner, Eric. *Vertical Heartland: A Rock Climber's Guide to Southern Illinois. 3rd edition.*
Buncombe, Illinois: Vertical Heartland.
   This is the definitive guide to the subject, covering not only where to climb but specific
   routes, ratings, and recommendations. Order from www.verticalheartland.com/Vertical
   Heartland.html

Wiggers, Raymond. *Geology Underfoot in Illinois.* Missoula, Montana: Mountain Press,
1997.
   Engaging and entertaining, this volume reads like a travel guidebook, presenting the
   geology of selected sites around the state and explaining why the hills, valleys, rivers,
   and canyons look the way they do.

WEBSITES

ADVENTURES WITH UNCLE BOB: www.illinois.sierraclub.org/shawnee/UncleBob/adventures.htm
Hiking guides, primarily for southern Illinois, from the Shawnee Group of the Sierra Club.

I FISH ILLINOIS: www.ifishillinois.org
The state's official fishing Web site. You'll find helpful information under "Places to Fish"
and "Family Fishing Hotspots," and the weekly fishing reports on specific waterways will
tell you what's biting and on what.

ILLINOIS HISTORIC SITES: www.illinoishistory.gov/hs/sites.htm
Official gateway to all state historic sites.

ILLINOIS STATE PARKS: www.dnr.state.il.us/lands/landmgt/parks/index.htm
Illinois Department of Natural Resources' gateway to all state parks and other recreation
areas.

SHAWNEE MOUNTAIN BIKE ASSOCIATION: www.smbatrails.com
Detailed trail maps and forums for finding current information on mountain biking in
and around the Shawnee National Forest.

SHAWNEE NATIONAL FOREST: www.fs.fed.us/r9/forests/shawnee
Home page of the Shawnee, which includes links to the most recent information about
closings, restrictions, and changes. Click on the "Interactive Map" link for a very helpful
overview of all trails and recreational venues throughout the forest.

APPENDIX B:
CAMPING-EQUIPMENT
CHECKLIST

Except for the large and bulky items on this list, I keep a plastic storage container full of the essentials for car camping so they're ready to go when I am. I make a last-minute check of the inventory, resupply anything that's low or missing, and away I go.

COOKING UTENSILS
Aluminum foil
Bottle opener
Can opener
Corkscrew
Cups, plastic or tin
Dish soap (biodegradable), sponge, and towel
Flatware
Frying pan
Fuel for stove
Matches in waterproof container
Plates
Pocketknife
Pot with lid
Salt, pepper, spices, sugar, cooking oil, and maple syrup in spillproof containers
Spatula
Stove
Wooden spoon

FIRST-AID KIT
Antibiotic cream
Band-Aids®
Diphenhydramine (Benadryl®)
Gauze pads
Ibuprofen or aspirin
Insect repellent
Lip balm
Moleskin®
Snakebite kit
Sunscreen
Tape, waterproof adhesive

SLEEPING GEAR
Pillow
Sleeping bag
Sleeping pad, inflatable or insulated
Tent with ground tarp and rainfly

MISCELLANEOUS
Bath soap (biodegradable), washcloth, and towel
Camp chair
Candles
Cooler
Deck of cards
Duct tape
Fire starter
Flashlight or headlamp with fresh batteries
Foul-weather clothing
Paper towels
Plastic zip-top bags
Sunglasses
Toilet paper
Water bottle
Wool or fleece blanket
Optional:
Barbecue grill
Binoculars
Field guides
Fishing rod and tackle
Hatchet
Kayak and related paddling gear
Lantern
Maps (road, topographic, trails, and so on)
Mountain bike and related riding gear

INDEX

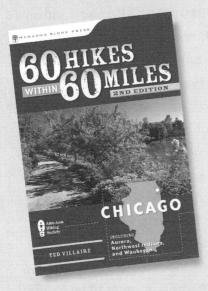
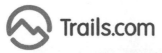